MOMENTS OF *Joy*

FIFTY-TWO IDEAS TO NURTURE
GREATER MEANING
FROM LIFE

MOMENTS OF Joy

FIFTY-TWO IDEAS TO NURTURE
GREATER MEANING
FROM LIFE

CHRIS BENTLEY

Copyright 2023 © Chris Bentley

All rights reserved. No part of this book may be reproduced in any form or by any electronic or mechanical means, including information and retrieval systems, without permission in writing from the publisher, except by reviewers, who may quote brief passages for review.

Paperback ISBN: 979-8-9850664-2-5

Library of Congress Control Number: 2023907562

To my family, who brings me countless joys

DEAR READER,

Please read this first! I know it's customary to skip the introductions of books, but I hope you'll indulge me this once.

Throughout my life, I've been drawn to the self-improvement sections within bookstores. I was the geeky twelve-year-old who talked about the elements of *How to Win Friends and Influence People* in his sixth-grade social studies class and sought relationship advice from books long before knowing how to shave.

I start this book by laying that on the table in order to explain that the self-improvement book genre has been very important to me. I hope that many of you have found comfort, peace, and advice from many great books, but eventually, I noticed that many a self-improvement book is built upon one insightful and clever concept that could fit on a napkin and that the rest of the couple hundred pages within said book are reiterations or elaborations on that simple thought.

So, when I went about writing this book, I wanted to take a different approach. This book is a collection of fifty-two vignettes—to correspond with the fifty-two weeks in a year. The vignettes contain my personal experiences, scientific studies, or life lessons. All the selections are purposefully brief and, hopefully, easily digested.

The book is also divided into four sections, corresponding to the four seasons of the year. But let me be clear: the book doesn't have to be read in any particular way, order, or timeline. The seasonal approach and the fifty-two-week selections are simply designed to help those readers who might enjoy reading the book a certain way.

To make your reading time as productive and useful as possible, here are a few ways to read it.

READ STRAIGHT THROUGH

This book is a collection of ideas, stories, and suggestions, so if you want to read them all at once rather than breaking the concepts into weekly or seasonal focuses, that's completely fine.

READ A SECTION PER WEEK

The fifty-two selections are designed to make it easier to focus on one concept, by allowing you the necessary time to practice the lessons learned one week at a time. By doing this, you will have a year's worth of things you can try in order to experience a bit more joy in your life.

You can also follow the prompts found on the online calendar provided on my website (www.chrisbentleyinc.com). The weekly prompts ask questions and offer suggestions. The online calendar can be downloaded for free as a printable PDF, so it can be hung up and used as a chronicle of your journey through the practices and concepts each selection covers. There is also plenty of space for you to write down your own questions or ideas that you want to focus on each week. So don't let my prompts deter you from personalizing the calendar in the way that will be most meaningful to you.

FOCUS ON ONE QUARTER OF THE YEAR AT A TIME

Since the book is divided into four sections, one for each of the four seasons of the year, you could read one section a quarter and choose a theme or a couple of concepts to focus on during that season. I offer a free online printable PDF form for that approach as well, under the *resources* heading at www.chrisbentleyinc.com. You can print it out and hang it up to be reminded of the life lessons you're trying to incorporate in your own life.

No matter how you decide to read this book, it is my sincere hope that reading it will bring at least a bit more joy and meaning into your life. I contemplated the ideas that make up this book during some of the darkest days of the COVID-19 pandemic. I drew such joy and hope from sharing the ideas with others through live-streaming sessions and individual blog posts that I felt as though I needed to share them with others who also went through that challenging time, as well as with those who may now face any number of other challenges that life throws at us.

Although I might not have the privilege to know all of you personally, please understand that with this book comes all of my well-wishes for peace, joy, and a meaningful life for you and those whom you love and care for.

Yours with hope,
Chris

CONTENTS

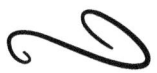

Spring

Using Ritual to Mark Our Days 3
The Marvels of Melding Musical Magic 7
Setting Up Our Seeds to Grow 11
Revitalizing Old Cherry Trees 15
Ebbing and Flowing Through the Punches 19
Jumpstarting Our Seedlings Again 23
Surprised by Poppies 27
Gratitude Even for the House Finches 29
Let's Focus on Our Own Game 33
Unyielding Firmness Through the Hardest Times 37
Pruning Back Before the Wind Storms 41
Having a Whale of an Impact One Person at a Time 45
Do What Is Expected and Then a Little Bit More 49

Summer

SINGING OUR SONG EVEN IF NO ONE IS LISTENING	55
PROVIDING SHADE FOR FUTURE GENERATIONS	57
BUILDING UPON THE SHOULDERS OF OTHER PEOPLE'S SANDCASTLES	61
TAKING CARE OF OURSELVES SETS US UP TO ASSIST OTHERS	65
BECOMING THE SHADE ON A HOT DAY	69
POTENTIAL IS A LOT LIKE A BOX OF ACORNS	73
MEETING PEOPLE WHERE THEY ARE	75
CLEAN OUT THAT WATERING CAN	79
IT'S A GRAND OLE COMPLICATED FLAG	81
CHANGING THE WORLD ONE MOMENT OF GENEROSITY AT A TIME	85
FORGED IN THE FIRES OF FRIENDSHIP & KINDNESS	89
WISDOM OF SHEEPDOGS	93
RUNNING TOWARD THE MORNING SUN	97
THAT DOG-EAT-DOG WORLD SHOULD JUST TAKE A BREATH	99

Fall

THE POWER OF ONE TOUCH IN OUR LIVES	105
THREE CHEERS FOR TEACHERS	109
PUDDLE HOPPING AND OTHER THRILLING PROSPECTS	113
THE GRAND ADVENTURE OF IMAGINING WHO WE WANT TO BE	117
SHOWING OUR TRUE COLORS	121
IF A TREE CHANGES COLOR IN THE WOODS, DO WE NOTICE?	123
WHAT HAPPENS AFTER THE CAR CRASH	125

REPLACING OUR TIRES TO AVOID THE WRECK. 129
EMBRACING THE RAINSTORMS WITH A GOOD PAIR OF RAIN BOOTS 133
LETTING OUR MISTAKES FLOW DOWN RIVER 137
WHAT THE WORLD NEEDS NOW - EMPATHY. 139
CELEBRATING AND HONORING THE COURAGE & SERVICE OF VETERANS 141
MODERN-DAY GOOD SAMARITANS 143

Winter

LET GO TO EMBRACE THE NEW. 149
DEATH BED GOAL SETTING 153
GATHER YE ROSEBUDS AND MAYBE STOP TO SMELL SOME TOO 157
HAPPY BROWN HOG DAY!. 161
JOY DURING THE RAINSTORMS 165
WE CAN LEARN A LOT FROM THE TREES 169
MINIMIZING MISSTEPS. 171
THE ELEGANCE OF CREAM SODA AND A PINK COOKIE 175
FILLING THE UNFORGIVING MINUTE WITH NURTURING SOIL & SUNLIGHT . . . 179
LEVERAGING HISTORY'S PERSPECTIVE 183
THE GIVING AND LIVING TREE 185
CHANGING OUR LIVES ONE HAIR CUT AT A TIME 189
HERE'S THE REAL DEAL ON NEW YEAR'S RESOLUTIONS 193
ENDNOTES: 197
ABOUT THE AUTHOR 199

Spring

USING RITUAL
TO MARK OUR DAYS

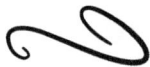

Whatever might speak to you, I hope you find a simple ritual that you can perform daily to help you say, "Yes, I lived this day."

Early in 2022, I started a ritual. Each day, I got a small peat pot out of a large stack that I keep in the corner of my kitchen and filled it with soil. I placed a tiny tree seed on top of the soil, covered it with a bit of additional soil, and added a gentle amount of water. Then I marked the pot with a plastic garden flag—the sort you see at your local nursery that identifies plant species. Each flag I stuck into a pot had the details of the type of tree I'd planted and what day I'd planted it. I kept the small pots in rows by a sunny window on a workshop shelf, and was thrilled to discover the first seedlings burst from the soil after about a month.

When I've told people about this particular ritual, their first response has usually been, "Where will you plant all of those trees when they grow?" and that was usually followed up with, "You're planting a tree *every day?*"

Each time, I do my best to explain that it'll be years until the trees are large enough to need much more space than they currently take up since they are oak and pine trees, which tend to be slower growing. And yes, I did this consistently for all of 2022, every morning, just before eating my breakfast.

This ritual holds added meaning for me because once the seeds are nestled in their pots, I take a minute or two to visualize the seeds. I imagine roots first breaking out of the seeds' shells and grasping hold of the nutrients in the soil. And I like to think about the joy of seeing the seeds sprout above the soil and experience sunlight for the first time. When I think about the growth of these seeds—all the immense potential that each has to become massive trees—I think about how I can grasp ahold of good things that can help me and others grow as well.

This was only one small (but significant for me) action that I took every day. It, as well as a couple of other rituals, including mindfulness exercises and writing in a gratitude journal every night, helps me to make better sense of and to mark my day.

So often over the last couple years, I'd felt like my days had melted together like a box of crayons left outside on the hot asphalt. Good things happened practically every day, but I realized I wasn't paying enough attention to those good things. There's nothing necessarily wrong with going with the flow, but I realized that I had been coasting from day to day without giving each day the kind of thanks it deserved. Marking each day with simple rituals has helped me break out of that coasting mode and get a bit closer to celebrating every day for its own merits.

Many people think rituals belong only in the realm of religion or spirituality. Rituals certainly don't have to be religious. In fact, I'd bet that, although we might not be conscious enough most days to call them *rituals*, our morning routines are very much just that. Do you flip on—or I guess more appropriately these days, ask Alexa to turn on—the radio to catch up on news while you're making and eating breakfast? Do you go for a jog, looking forward to listening to a favorite podcast or audiobook?

Using the word *ritual* to refer to these morning routines matters. What we call something can either become commonplace or approach sacredness, depending on how we choose to look at our actions. What happens when things once considered routines or habits become important rituals? The very same actions take on completely new and inspiring meaning.

Simple rituals can make even the hardest of circumstances a bit more bearable. I recall visiting a dear elderly neighbor who was nearing the end of his life, as well as his wife, who visited him daily in the hospital. On one particular occasion, I noticed a friendly, leafy, green plant propped up on the windowsill that seemed to be doing very well. My neighbor's wife told me that she gave the plant a little drink each morning when she visited her husband. She first took care of the plant because her husband had always loved gardening, but in time, it mostly gave her a way to make things a bit better for her husband. She also recognized that her husband was wavering in and out of consciousness at the time, so it had become important for her too.

So where does the added meaning and sense of connection come from?

Meaning and connection come, in part, from the power of ritual. We choose to label a routine as a ritual. We choose to go through those rituals even when (maybe especially when) we don't feel like it. The true power of ritual comes when we are willing to perform the action even when we aren't super excited to do so. Then, when we are on the other side of those harder times, we have a new sense of connection to our rituals and a greater appreciation for their balancing effect, making it easier to perform them in the future.

Maybe planting trees isn't your thing. But whatever your thing may be, I hope you find a simple ritual that you can perform daily to help you say, "Yes, I lived this day."

THE MARVELS OF MELDING MUSICAL MAGIC

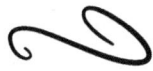

We are all human and, as such, our greatest accomplishments come when we work together.

I remember when I had my first musical theater experience. I was a freshman in high school. Just a kid really. We were putting on *Anything Goes,* which is a large musical in about every sense. The director was rather legendary, and I was thrilled to be a chorus member in her production. But there were certainly plenty of moments when I questioned why in the world I had agreed to participate in such a crazy thing.

One particular afternoon, a small group was practicing choreography at the same time that there were two or three other groups practicing their entrances for the opening number while several of the leads were practicing there speaking and acting roles.

Musicals generally have a story line as well as great songs, so there's some acting and regular speech thrown in among all the singing and dancing.

All of that was going on at the same time that the stage crew was setting the lighting and working on the set. So we had hammers banging on wood scaffolding, lights fading off and on, dozens of voices either singing or speaking with their theatrical voices (i.e. loudly). There was so much coming and going and such a buzz of activity that if someone wasn't aware that it was a musical rehearsal, they would have been quite alarmed.

And yet, despite all the chaos, somehow or other, all the pieces came together, and I was proud to be a part of the finished product, which offered, after several months of practice, four or five performances. But that didn't matter for some reason. For nearly half of the school year, I was tied to this group of singing performers in order to put on a few performances. And though it was fun to perform for an audience and to hear the kind things family and friends said about the production, hands-down, the thing that made it all worthwhile was the sense of community that I felt as a result of participating in the production—participating in something so much bigger and grander than me.

Humans are very much social animals. I know that some of us are more extroverted than others, but all of us rely on our own circles of community to gain validation, to learn to be a successful citizen and member of our community, and to learn what it feels like to be loved and to love others. It's remarkable to think of all the people who work behind the scenes of our lives, who bring so much richness and meaning to our lives. I think back on the profound experiences that I had in college and have in my faith community. I think of the times I've helped out with city events and serving (in my own small ways) in my local community. All of these experiences came about because I participated in and was a part of something larger than myself, something with intricacies that I still don't fully understand.

By being part of large productions like *Anything Goes*, we also learn to navigate differences in new ways. There are different political affiliations, hobbies, life experiences, economic circumstances, clothing styles, and so much more all meshed into this microcosm of humanity. But through such productions we are able to work together because we focus on the common goal of putting on the best production that we possibly can. This isn't to say that we care any less about all of those other things, but we are given a chance to get to know and like each other based on the many other pieces of who we are.

It takes a lot of time and dedication, while sometimes enduring harsh criticism, to pull off even as much as a high school musical. But all of that work and time is worth it. The sense of accomplishment that comes from, not only learning to sing and dance, but also from the reminder that we are all human and, as such, our greatest accomplishments come when we are willing to get to know others more holistically and work together for a common cause.

SETTING UP OUR SEEDS TO GROW

Becoming who we want to become depends
on our building upon keystone habits
and then giving ourselves enough space
and time to do them consistently.

We all are familiar with the steps of growing seeds. Assuming that the seeds are viable—meaning capable of growing—the steps are quite simple:

1. Get a container.

2. Fill the container with nutrient-rich soil.

3. Place the seed near the top of the soil and cover with more soil.

4. Water frequently.

That's basically it.

Once the seed sprouts, make sure it gets regular sun and water. After that, you'll pretty much have a successfully growing seedling. There are obviously some more delicate varieties of seedlings—ones that only grow in soil with a certain acidity or temperature or in full sunlight. But as a basic set of principles, that's really it, as far as growing a seedling goes.

Still, we need to do all of those things to be successful. If we have the best soil but never water our seed, it doesn't matter how rich of an environment we placed it in; the seed won't grow. The same is true if we have a great soil base and have a good habit of watering it frequently; if we don't plant the seed, nothing will ever grow (except for some potential weeds).

There are also some life situations and experiences that do not require us to perform all the steps; doing less is perfectly acceptable. Of course, there are also a lot of situations in life that aren't as straight forward as planting and growing seeds.

But there are some situations where we can't cut corners—we can't do some of the steps while we ignore others. There are many ways to stay healthy, and we can practice several of them, but if we struggle to get enough sleep, a viscous cycle starts, and that leads to bad outcomes every time. We might want to learn a language, so we buy the language program and books and plan a trip to visit the country where that language is spoken, but if we never practice speaking the language, we're going to have a hard time learning to speak it in any practical way.

It's important that we find out what keystone behaviors are vital to helping us become who we want to become and then make sure that we give ourselves sufficient space and time to consistently practice those behaviors. The keystone behaviors will be different for everyone, but you can discover yours by watching for activities that help you make better decisions.

> **Keystone behaviors are behaviors that provide a multiplier effect, causing small amounts of action to lead to a big positive change.**

A common keystone behavior is exercising first thing in the morning. By exercising when we first wake up, the possibility that we will make better dietary choices goes up, which in turn, will lead to higher levels of energy during the day and might lead to greater task accomplishments that will lead to a greater sense of well-being and achievement. Another keystone behavior to try might be taking ten minutes a day for mindfulness. Doing that could lead to having a greater ability to deal with regular frustrations in ways that help strengthen relationships and lower stress levels.

Generally, starting small and then growing, based on incremental improvements, is a more sustainable way of carving time and space as we incorporate these powerful behaviors.

When I was training for my first marathon, the prospect of running a full 26.2-mile marathon was far too much for me to think about. Instead, I gladly focused on the two-mile run I scheduled those first few days of training. Then, gradually, I added mileage.

And I'd dare say, there are a few sure-fire ways to impede our hope and meaning in life, even if we are doing a lot of good things. Dwelling on regret throughout the day, focusing so much on others' needs but never on our own, expecting the next achievement to completely fill our fulfillment bucket without being clear of what we really value or care about…

To avoid these pitfalls, we can't do the same thing we normally do and expect a different result. Similar to making small time adjustments to take healthier actions, we can make incremental changes to our thought process throughout the day. If our usual paradigm includes worrying about the future, each day, we can intentionally schedule small bursts of time to focus on things that excite us about the future, or even better, focus on things that excite us that day.

**Keeping a daily gratitude journal is a great way
to focus your mind on the good around you.**

There are so many good things that we can be involved in, and we absolutely should take advantage of such opportunities. Among all the good things we can be a part of, though, it is also vital that we discover our own needs and what brings meaning and hope to each of us, individually, and then remember to plant our seeds and water them so they can grow.

REVITALIZING OLD CHERRY TREES

We are worthy of love and support even if we don't feel up to everything that life expects of us. Carving out a few moments of our day to nourish and trim back the excesses in our lives can lead us to bear wholesome and delicious fruit.

While I was working on my undergraduate degree at Weber State University, I had many wonderful opportunities to support and organize projects in areas that I was not an expert in but that I felt were important.

One of those tangential passion projects was a push to break the Guinness world record for the most trees planted within an hour. A somewhat obscure record, for sure, but there is a reason why those annual books are a thousand pages with a six-point font size. In any case, the record was more of a catalyst than the underlying goal, which was actually to just plant a bunch of trees.

One area of campus that the university botanist, Dr. Gatherum, identified as a potential gold mine of tree-planting possibilities was on the outskirts of campus behind some annex houses that had been converted into offices. Dr. Gatherum and I worked with some of his students to layout a design for his own passion project: the development of a community orchard.

We would plant twenty-five fruit trees, a mix of apple, pear, plum, and peach. I even won funding through a special grant to purchase the trees. In order to reach our 135 tree-planting goal, other planting locations were scattered throughout the campus and even in surrounding cities.

The day of the grand tree-planting event arrived, and I rallied the troops at the main plaza bell tower and then sent them out to their respective planting locations. At that point, I coordinated the start time, which was at the strike of noon. I immediately called all the planting captains and told them we were a go.

All said and done, within an hour, we'd planted 135 trees, breaking the old record by more than double. We even got affidavits signed by the university president and the mayors of the two cities where trees were planted in coordination with their city park departments. That was a very exciting day!

I suppose there are many lessons that could be drawn from such an experience. But as I recently considered it, I was reminded of something entirely different that was connected to that experience.

The first time Dr. Gatherum and I walked the grounds where we would plant twenty-five fruit trees, it became quite obvious why the professor would want to plant fruit trees in that particular location. In the backyards of the two annex university buildings, stood two tired, gnarled cherry trees and an overgrown apple tree.

I was fascinated because, although it was clearly the time of the year when those old fruit trees should have been blossoming, I didn't see a single blossom anywhere. Puzzled, I asked Dr. Gatherum what was going on. "Are the trees dying," I wondered?

He explained the trees were quite healthy, but that it had been so long since they had been pruned or fertilized that the trees had slowly reverted to just putting up leaves. "To have fruit trees bear a lot of fruit," he continued, "we have to do some care for the trees. The trees will give to us, if we give to the trees." Dr. Gatherum was hoping to incorporate the new twenty-five fruit trees, along with the older three, into a new course on orchard maintenance in the botany department. And in that way, those three tired trees could get the care they needed to be productive while also being joined by several new trees. Collectively, all the trees could have new purpose.

I've reflected back on that experience and that particular interaction many times over the years. An apple tree is still an apple tree even if it's currently not bearing fruit. And in a similar way, we are very much still worthy of love and support, even if we don't feel up to everything that life expects out of us. And isn't it such a hopeful thought—that carving out a few moments out of our day to nourish our bodies and minds and prune back the excesses in our lives can lead us to bearing such wholesome and delicious fruit, just like the students at the university did for those old, tired trees.

EBBING AND FLOWING THROUGH THE PUNCHES

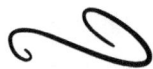

The ocean waves have ebbed and flowed every day for billions of years. It reminds us that we'll make it through even the hardest times.

I had a lot of health challenges as a kid, including a brain injury caused by a cerebral arterial venous malformation (AVM) that required eight surgeries and decades' worth of therapy. While I'm so grateful for the abilities I've been able to regain, there are still unique challenges that I face every day because of that brain injury.

I remember a moment when I was in the hospital after my eighth and, thankfully, final brain surgery. At that moment, I'd lost the ability to talk with no clear indication of when I would regain that ability, if ever. I was thinking that night about what some of my high school classmates might be doing in that moment, rather than lying in a hospital bed trying to figure out how to take the AP Literature test without the ability to read. They hadn't lost that ability due to the resection of a portion of their brains like I had during that last surgery.

Slowly, over the next several months, I started to regain the abilities I'd lost. I focused on speech and physical therapy weekly. And while I struggled to read a single page of *Harry Potter* in less than twenty minutes, I gradually picked up speed. I also built up my physical stamina by taking daily walks and short bike rides that I slowly stretched to a few miles. Then a few years later, I gratefully completed my first marathon.

As I look back at those daily struggles, I recognize two key insights that helped me make it through those first few months of recovery. First, I needed to focus on the daily micro-improvements. I did this by keeping track of my progress, whether that was my minutes-per-page reading speed or the distance I walked. I also had to recognize how counterproductive longing for the time before that last surgery really was. Instead of dwelling on how good things used to be, I focused on my gratitude that the AVM was gone and that I no longer ran the risk of having to go through that procedure again.

The stretch of any one ocean wave doesn't tell us whether the tide is coming in, going out, or how far the high tide might reach at its full extent. We can only determine that by taking note over time and marking its progress. One day's improvement might seem so miniscule, but if we measure our progress over a week or month, we will likely be amazed at how far we have come.

One might say I have some sense of how impossible certain tasks can seem. But something I learn from watching ocean waves is that, without fail, they still wash up against the beach. They still rise and fall with the tides. And they still leave me willing, calmer, and more hopeful.

I survived that night, and I eventually relearned how to talk and read. I took and passed that AP Literature test, which I am so grateful for. But sometimes we aren't quite that fortunate. Sometimes we have to deal with disappointments as well as misfortune. Those times are the true tests of our endurance and hope. And though we might have to just grit our teeth and push through, once we come out on the other side, we know that we are capable of doing incredibly hard things. And that is a valuable thing to recognize about ourselves.

We can always look to the next morning. We can always hope and work toward good things as we deal with those ebbs and flows of life. And we can always cling to those good moments that come each day. As we do that, somehow, the morning sunlight of the next day shines all the brighter.

JUMPSTARTING OUR SEEDLINGS AGAIN

When we make the decision to dump the bad soil from our seedling pots and replant seeds with fresh, new soil, not only are we likelier to have seedlings sprout, but we become wiser.

As a new daily ritual and a way to mark each day, I planted one tree seed each morning throughout 2022. After the ninetieth day of planting a single tree seed in a peat pot, I made a discovery—several of the seeds were sprouting by then, but not the ones I expected. The first forty or so seeds weren't growing, even after three months of care.

My first impulse was to give the seeds a bit more time. *Surely they'll sprout soon, and if I toss them out and start over with new seeds, all that potential effort that those seeds have gone through will be wasted,* I thought.

I deliberated on what to do for a few days, and I came to a conclusion. Since I had planted the same sort of seeds in the early batches that I had planted with later plantings, and since my watering schedules and the amount of sunlight were the same, the soil quality must have been problem.

Germinating seeds are pretty vulnerable to their growing environments. Conditions have to be pretty darn good or else the seeds just won't grow. And the ground in which the seeds are planted is clearly one of, if not the most important factor. How often do we assume that dirt is dirt and that once we've filled a pot with some type of earth, we can jump directly into the daily grind of watering the seeds? Surely, any type of soil will do, right? I've found that to be very untrue.

In a similar way, I've come to realize that certain aspects of my life fit into the same sort of false assumption. We don't always make sure that our goals are grounded in the firmest and richest soils. Perhaps some nights we stay up too late and then regret it the next morning. Do we promise ourselves to get to bed by 10:30 p.m. each night? Unless we set a reminder at 10:00 p.m., giving us time to start our bedtime routines and transition from our current activities, inevitably, we'll start our bedtime routines late, which means we won't meet our goals.

Economists talk about something called the sunk-cost fallacy. In a nutshell, the fallacy describes faulty logic that we humans fall for. We continue to invest in causes, goals, projects, businesses, and other initiatives rather than cut bait and try something else. In essence, it's that old belief that *we've already come this far, we might as well keep going.* I definitely faced this fallacy when deciding what to do with the dozens of pots that weren't sprouting. Should I empty the pots, get better soil, and replant, or should I wait for seeds planted in poor soil to somehow beat the odds and start growing?

Determining whether to adjust our goal and direction is not an easy decision to make. Sometimes the alternative isn't nearly as cut and dried as the economic graphs in the typical Economics 101 course would lead us to believe. Sometimes we've invested a considerable amount of emotional connection and a portion of our personal identities into our initiatives. We might worry about what others might think of us if we change course, especially after having declared our intentions to friends, family, or our social media connections.

But when we determine it's the best course of action to, metaphorically speaking, dump the bad soil from our seedling pots and replant seeds with fresh, new soil, not only are we likelier to have the kind of outcomes we set out to have in the first place, but we're also better for having experienced disappointments. Now we know how to avoid such setbacks. And, of course, there is a happy ending to my potted seed story. Several weeks after replacing the soil in the pots, rows of thriving seedlings burst above the better soil.

SURPRISED BY POPPIES

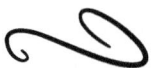

Beautiful and surprising things are happening all around us if we slow down enough to see them.

I drove past a massive industrial park one early spring day. It was one of those classic, hulking complexes of cold concrete and endless parking lots that surround impossibly long, uniform structures made up of rows of long concrete buildings. Growing up, I had a business depot with the same look and feel, and as I've traveled around the country, I've seen the same setup in most mid- to-large-sized towns.

Just before I was about to disregard the complex entirely, as we tend to do when driving in familiar territories, something struck my eye: bright-orange flecks were scattered around what I assumed to be a field of weeds. At first, I assumed the specks were bits of plastic or soda cans tossed and disregarded by the maintenance folks running the facilities. I even imagined one of the maintenance workers joking with a coworker: "Come on! The stuff that goes on inside is what really matters. They don't make money by making their yard look nice." But then I recognized those bright-colored specks that were popping up above the grass that could have used a mow.

It was a field of bright-orange poppies that filled the hillside. As I drove past, I could make out their rich purple centers and their irreverently psychedelic, bright petals. They were absolutely stunning. I imagine they had grown spontaneously due to birds or the wind picking up the seeds from some garden nearby and dropping them on the verdant ground that—during this time of the year, in Oregon, with the amount of rain and mild temperatures—can grow just about anything.

It was only a moment really. I was past the field of poppies too soon, and I fought the urge to jump out of the car in the middle of traffic to get a better look. But it definitely taught me an important lesson: beautiful and surprising things are happening all around us if we slow down enough to see them.

These small and beautiful moments can add up to a lot of richness in our lives if we watch for them each day. We might find them in the delighted sound of a child's laugh as they skip past on the street. We might discover one with a family member as we spend an extra minute or two with them, completely present in the moment. Or a birdsong might strike our ears, and we might stop to listen closer when the song sounds again.

GRATITUDE EVEN FOR THE HOUSE FINCHES

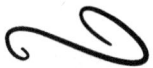

> We collectively gain so much more than any one of us pays into society. When we're grateful for the hidden contributions of unsung contributors, our gratitude sings within our souls.

I'm absolutely blown away by bird migrations. I love seeing the migratory birds returning north this time of the year. Take the Arctic Tern for example. They travel from practically one pole to the other twice a year, or roughly fifty-five thousand miles per year. And according to Bird Life International, since they can live up to thirty years, their migration patterns can mean traveling the same distance to the moon and back three times in one Arctic Tern's lifetime, or almost 1.5 million miles, or over fifty-seven times around the Earth![1]

Many migratory birds make remarkable attempts to follow their instincts and their chemical triggers to pass on their genetic code for future generations. It's easy to anthropomorphize the valiant attempts of protecting their single eggs when watching documentaries like the *March of the Penguins* because their work ethic and sacrifice reaches heroic levels. I don't know what feelings or emotions drive these amazing animals to do such remarkable feats, but there are many poignant lessons that we can draw from the examples set by the animal kingdom.

The thing that has struck me most as I've seen house finches, larks, and warblers come back from their distant travels is how little notice and appreciation I give to the birdsongs that often wake me up in the morning. Is there a more pleasant alarm clock then birdsong? We can easily overlook the extraordinary efforts the birds that sing in our backyards have taken in order to sing in our neighborhoods if we choose to.

It's easy to assume that the sparrows and robins will return year after year because that's nature's way and we don't do anything to make it happen. They just show up come spring. With things that automatically bring us satisfaction, comfort, and joy that we haven't earned and don't necessarily deserve, we don't need to intercede. We could support an organization that assists migratory birds. But it's not like any one of us could teach a whole species a better way to migrate. But we can be grateful for the unearned gifts. Nature provides many other unearned gifts that are easily overlooked as well. A beautiful sunset. A cool breeze during a morning jog. A rainbow piercing a gray sky. Even a tree seedling growing.

There are also many examples in our own species' interdependence. Remember early on in the COVID-19 pandemic when toilet paper and hand sanitizer were hard to find, and grocery store shelves were unusually bare of items that we expect to always be available?

It's incredible to think of the hundreds of people who put effort into producing the products that end up on grocery store shelves—people who, most of the time, get no attention or credit for their work. And there are so many other unsung contributors: the public-works people who clean our gutters and plow our streets and pick up our garbage every week. The podcast creators or radio producers who create entertaining content that transforms an otherwise-dreary commute to work into an engaging experience. The public artists who beautify our city parks. Modern society relies on these people to show up and do their jobs, and our lives are made better every day because they do.

Although we can say they get paid to do their jobs, we don't directly pay their salaries. We might contribute a tiny fraction of their pay by buying products or paying taxes, but collectively, we gain much more than any one person pays into society for these benefits—benefits that make our lives more comfortable, safe, and enjoyable. And just like the migratory birds, we don't have to contribute more than what we already do, but there is something soul-enriching in recognizing and being grateful for their efforts. So maybe the next time we go to the grocery store, we can give a genuine smile and offer a little thank you to the clerk stocking the shelves, or the next time we're taking a walk in the neighborhood park we can wave at the landscaping crew. It doesn't cost us anything to be grateful, and we might be surprised at how enriching it is to send that gratitude into the world.

LET'S FOCUS ON OUR OWN GAME

We can build trust in our friends and family by showing that we trust them. As we do that, they are likelier to look to us for listening ears, gentle nudges, and simple suggestions.

A while back, I played Chinese Checkers with a few dear friends. It had been decades since I'd last played that game, so, if you, like me, haven't played it for a while, let me walk you through the very simple objective and rules.

Each player picks a certain color of marble and sets up their base in a triangle formation right in front of where they're sitting, kind of like an upside-down bowling-pin setup. Then each player takes turns moving one marble at a time with the goal of getting all of their marbles across the board to the opposite triangle bowling-bin base.

It seems very simple, but you can imagine how complex it can get in the middle of the board when four-or-so players all charge ahead from different directions. And, if you butt up against an opponent's marble and there is an open hole on the other side of said marble, you can jump over it. Moreover, so long as that condition continues to exist, you can jump multiple marbles. This can move your marbles toward their target home base quickly, if you use the right strategy.

By the end of the first game, I was comfortable with the game play, but the first few turns of the next game, I took my time and carefully weighed my options. Meanwhile, my three friends rather unhelpfully would expound with sighs and *oohs* periodically followed by "Oh my goodness! I see a really great move for you! I hope you see it!"

I tried my best to take their comments as good-hearted and spontaneous outbursts that spurred from the intensity and excitement of the game, but a curious thing happened almost every time I finished my turn. My friends would compliment my move and then say to some effect that there was a better move. As they said this, they would try to show me how their move would have been better than the one I had made. Except, almost without fail, when they tried playing out the move, it would end up being illegal or not being nearly as good as their *oohs* and *ahhs* implied.

It made me laugh while playing the game, but since then, I've reflected on how easy it is to assume that we know what is best for our friends and family members. How often does the thought pop into our heads that our sister would be better off if she would get out of that relationship? Or that our best friend would feel more excitement for life and break free of their current depression if they left the house more?

If we look back on the past few weeks' worth of conversations, I bet we'd all discover that such thoughts have crept into our minds. We'd find that we say, "Ooh! I see the perfect move for you! I hope you see it!" and that, sometimes, we even share our game-plan corrections for our friends and family members with them. And if they decide not to take us up on our chosen game plan, sometimes we feel hurt.

But this is the thing: we will never be able to scrutinize anyone else's life better than they already do. Our perspective, though well-meaning and possibly based on meaningful past experiences, is just that—our perspective. Every other human being among the seven-plus billion of us, has his or her own game plan, and each of us has our eyes firmly placed on the next few moves to help ourselves advance to our home base.

Does that mean we should just leave people alone to fend for themselves in the world? No! But it does mean that we need to take a different tactic when we offer help. We can listen more than we share advice. We can build trust by showing our friends and family that we trust them. And we can show that we care about them regardless of what move they take. As we do that, they are likelier to look to us for listening ears, gentle nudges, and simple suggestions. And, in turn, we can remind ourselves that most of the "brilliant" moves we see for our friends aren't quite as brilliant, because those moves aren't ours to make.

UNYIELDING FIRMNESS THROUGH THE HARDEST TIMES

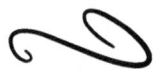

Don't put on a mask of smiles to hide the anguish you feel in your worst moments. Commit to pushing through. Continue the breathing and eating and sleeping that your body requires until you're able to start your climb out from the depths.

I remember the moment so distinctly. I had undergone my seventh brain surgery—which had gone really well, all things considered. Of course, no day that we have our head cut open is exactly a bluebird-on-my-shoulder kind of day, but things had gone according to plan, and I woke up from the anesthesia in a gentle enough way.

But the second operation of that hospital stay was a different story. I had been told that this surgery had been a success as well, but this time, I was wrenched out of the anesthesia with a jolt. Severe biting pain racked my head and neck. I felt very unsettled. And, worse still, I couldn't talk. I watched the nurses bustling past, attending to the many other patients in the unit. I tried to free my arms so that I could at least flag one down and maybe pantomime what I needed, but my arms were full of IVs, and I had tubes running to half a dozen different machines.

> **I hope that very few of us ever experience such a soul-crushing experience. To lose the ability to speak is startling to say the least, but in my case, I had already experienced it, and I knew how much time and effort relearning to speak could take. I also lost that ability when my initial brain injury occurred eight years before.**

So, I was lying in the ICU bed with a very thin sheet covering me, shivering silently, but desperately trying to get the attention of a nurse so I could at least get a decent blanket.

It is difficult to explain how excruciating it is to know what you want to say, but be unable to work the mechanics of your vocal cords, tongue, and mouth in conjunction with the right neural pathways to get those words out. It felt like my body was a foreign object—a piece of machinery I had never worked with before. Except, I absolutely knew I had been very good at operating that piece of machinery the day before.

Through painstaking effort, I finally blurted out the words "I'm cold" and "I can't talk." A nurse eventually understood what I was saying and got me a blanket. Rather than feeling better about myself at finally being understood, my alarm grew because I already knew the long road I had in front of me to regain those lost skills.

In time, I physically recovered enough from my surgeries that I could be discharged from the hospital. Relearning how to talk was a definite challenge, especially because I was a junior in high school at the time and was trying to prepare college applications and take ACT, SAT and AP tests. Being unable to talk coupled with the fact that I had to relearn how to read, definitely complicated things, to say the least. The last semester of my junior year, my teachers kindly sent me homework assignments that they probably assumed were the right difficulty level. My AP Literature teacher sent short stories rather than assigning novels. My U.S. History teacher sent study guides rather than requiring me to read whole chapters of the textbook. But even those stripped-down assignments were serious challenges for me. It took me hours to read even a couple of pages. My head still pounded severely, and that made it tough to focus on study guides.

I worked with a speech therapist weekly and had to learn new strategies for reading: an activity I've loved my whole life. The section of my head that the surgeons had opened impacted my vision as well, so I had to learn to scan a bit further to the right for the last few words when I came to what looked like the end of a page because that part of my visual field had been impacted. But we as humans do our best to get by and seek improvements, little by little, each day. And now, I love reading as much as I did before the surgery, and I probably talk more than a lot of my coworkers or friends think is good for me.

When we're in the thick of hard times, when we can't think of any possible way that life could ever hold joy for us again, when we wonder what good hope is because we don't believe that better days are possible—in those moments, we often struggle to believe we'll make it through. We doubt the truth that others say about our strength. We doubt that we could inspire anyone. That's when we need those superhuman reserves of fortitude.

One of the root meanings of the word fortitude stems from the Latin word for firmness. Isn't that a great goal for us to strive for during our worst moments? We don't have to put on a mask of smiles in an attempt to hide the actual anguish we feel. But we can commit ourselves to pushing through—to continue the breathing and eating and sleeping that our bodies require—until we're able to start our climb out from the depths. It is completely acceptable in these moments of heartache or loss or extreme challenge to not be okay.

We gain our reserves of firmness by developing discipline drop by drop. Doing small things over time can add up to making significant changes. Going to bed at a decent hour, setting an alarm at night and getting up when we know we should get up, eating as healthy as we can, taking moments to breathe and be present even for thirty seconds a couple of times a day. Deciding what you want to accomplish in the morning and not losing sight of that throughout the day. These small and simple things build up our reserve, so when we face these unimaginable obstacles, we can still draw on those reserves.

PRUNING BACK BEFORE THE WIND STORMS

Just like a tree with heavy, long branches in a windstorm, we are susceptible of heading down unhealthy roads if we don't prune away everything but what matters most.

On a bright morning in early spring, I was enjoying some sunshine out on my third-story balcony when I was surprised by a tree pruner cutting a large branch from a city tree growing at my eye level. After getting over the initial surprise (let's face it, I don't often have visitors at my third-story balcony) I jumped to the railing to watch.

A man was using a very impressive long-reach pruner to trim the trees downtown. Many of the branches were significant in size and easily a couple of inches in diameter. I was a little sad to say goodbye to the branches that had so nicely provided shade and a wonderful ambiance with a slight rustling of wind between their leaves.

Why do we prune trees?

Right after a tree has received a thorough pruning, it tends to look awkward for a few months, sometimes flat out ugly. That is counter to our primary goal for planting trees in the first place, right? We typically plant trees in hopes that they will grow strong and tall and provide a lot of great shade or fruit. We don't plant trees to thwart their growth or make them look as though they come from Ichabod Crane's dark forest.

I grew up in an area of Utah between two major canyons, and those canyons act like huge wind tunnels to funnel and focus wind velocity, especially in the early spring. When I was a child, the wind would sometimes whip through those canyons at sixty or seventy miles per hour. In fact, there were a couple of days when I would walk to school and lean into the wind only to be held in place despite using my entire body weight in an attempt to move forward. Those days, I watched even great, old trees sway violently.

I never really thought of those massive trees as being impacted by the wind. Their roots went down so deep that I assumed trees that had survived for sixty years had the ability to withstand wind storms. Surely they had seen worse wind storms than the ones I grew up dealing with. So it was a huge surprise when I walked outside one morning to see that an enormous birch tree at a neighbor's house had lost its most significant branch, leaving a gaping wound in its trunk that oozed sticky fluids.

The neighbors hired an arborist to see if they could save the tree, but ultimately, it was determined that the wound was just too big and that the tree was too much of a risk to the house. It had become more susceptible to disease and insects, which would weaken the tree even more and could cause it to blow over onto the house. With consistent pruning throughout its life, the tree may not have lost its branch and my neighbors may not have lost their tree. That's the purpose of pruning. It removes the heaviness of excess, allowing for movement and growth.

And isn't pruning the excess exactly what we need to do to remain healthy and strong ourselves? There are so many demands on our time and for our attention—a lot of which are worthwhile and matter a lot to us. It can be painful to prune back those activities or organizations or people or uses of our time and attention. But just like a tree with heavy, long branches is in danger of losing its limbs and risks being uprooted when the winds come, we are susceptible of heading down unhealthy roads if we don't decide what matters most. We must focus our attention on the most important people and activities in our lives.

Times will come when we need to prune away those worthwhile activities that aren't the best fit. If we can do that sometimes painful but necessary work, we will become stronger and healthier, and we will also be in a better situation to do what matters most. Moreover, when the winds of stress or fear or pain hit us, we'll be better able to withstand it because our lives will be better focused and well grounded.

HAVING A WHALE OF AN IMPACT ONE PERSON AT A TIME

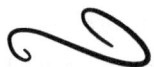

We never know our full impact, so let's try our best to share our truths with authenticity and conviction and not worry too much about the outcome.

I listened to a wonderful story on the radio a while back that commemorated the fiftieth anniversary of a humpback whale recording that became incredibly popular. The recording has been credited as a driving factor behind the interest in protecting whales and continues to have a huge impact in the way that we interact with whales today.

The story started with a naturalist who heard about a whale that had washed up on shore. The dead whale had been defaced rather horribly. People had carved initials into the body, and someone had stuck a cigarette butt in the whale's blowhole. The naturalist decided that he had to do something, but he didn't know what would be most impactful.

Then one day, rather randomly, a friend of his who worked with the U.S. Navy gave him an idea. The sailor told the naturalist about some sounds that he had recorded and believed were humpback whales. The naturalist went on board the ship and listened to the recording. In that moment, he talked about how haunting and heartbreaking the sounds were and how he felt confident that he had found his way of impacting the world. And I guess the rest, as they say, is history.[2]

But I've never been satisfied with the phrase "and the rest is history." It's easy to see how a certain series of events can lead up to remarkable results when we look back at it retroactively. It's much more difficult to believe in our actions and convictions when we are just living day by day, hoping that our impact will reach the people we're trying to reach. Undoubtedly, there had been thousands of attempts to influence society to care about whales that didn't have nearly as much of an impact. This particular naturalist might have dreamed of having this kind of impact, but he never could have known what kind of impact that recording would have over the coming decades. That gives me hope—seeing that even the most impactful decisions and programs are never sure things, and the people pushing their ideas through can never be certain what kind of impact will be had, or if they'll have an impact at all. What do we do with that? Does that mean we shouldn't try to make any impact?

I think a lot of us have aspirations of hitting it big with YouTube channels or becoming a known TikTok personality, but the reality is that most accounts get lost in the static. And, in reality, having many friends that have developed large followings on social media has shown me that it takes a lot of work to develop a big following. We shouldn't throw up our hands, deciding it's not worth trying to make an impact for good, but it is healthy to evaluate why we endeavor to make an impact.

If we endeavor for fame, disappoint and discouragement are easy to find when our goal isn't reached. On the other hand, if we aspire to make a contribution to the world and do our best to reach as many people as we can with an authentic and caring voice about an issue that matters to us, then the few people who start to follow our content can be impacted in significant ways. Indeed, we can feel fulfillment in that. And if we tell our story more times than might be easy or convenient, we are more likely to reach a larger audience than if we give up too early.

The naturalist who recorded and publicized those whale sounds was only trying to influence a few people to care more about whales. Instead, he ended up causing a worldwide environmental movement. We never know our full impact, so let's try our best to share our truths with authenticity and conviction and not worry too much about the outcome.

DO WHAT IS EXPECTED AND THEN A LITTLE BIT MORE

Do what is expected. Grease the gears and pump up the tires, but then do just ten percent more to show it matters. The reward for that ten percent addition can be profound.

I remember seeing my road bike right after its first tune-up done by the most conscientious bike shop. At the time, there were two bike shops in the town where I lived, and the other one always did acceptable work. They cleaned the gears and lubricated the derailleur and ensured proper air pressure for the tires. But the conscientious bike shop—they took such matters as personal calling. They cleaned the bike inside and out. They rewrapped the handle bars. My breaks never felt so secure or so consistent as they did after that shop worked on them. When I went to pick up my bike, the owner always had me sit on it to ensure proper height, and then he adjust the seat height and tweaked the handlebar angle to ensure a great fit.

Why would the conscientious shop go to such lengths to do such an exceptional job? I doubt very many of their customers knew to appreciate all the remarkable steps the bike mechanics went through to make the bikes not just function well, but wow their riders. After a couple of tune-ups, I started to feel like the shop was as dedicated to my bike enjoyment as I was, maybe more.

When I look out at my broader life experience, I see individuals who just do a task a bit more completely, more thoughtfully, and with more dedication than the rest of the crowd. My favorite teachers tended to be that way. I'm still connected with my elementary school librarian in large part because she was that way. Grocery store clerks, farmer's market shop owners, church leaders—there are so many.

And when I look at what they do differently that makes them stand out above the crowd, it becomes evident that they pay attention to the little details. They take the extra thirty seconds to lock my name into their memories so they can greet me in a personal way. They also tend to care a bit more about their work, the people they serve, and the impact they have within their communities.

> **I'm sure those who go the extra ten percent get paid the same with or without knowing my name or checking my seat height, but it sure changes the experience for me. In the end, I find I am more loyal to the store and more excited to visit the library. It becomes enjoyable to patronize the businesses and organizations run by these amazing individuals.**

When we recognize people who are willing to go beyond what is expected, we celebrate them and their efforts. How deeply we need people who care in our communities! And the best way to ensure that people like these persist is to try to become like them. So give it a try. Do what is expected, grease the gears and pump up the tires, but then do just ten percent more to show it matters. It doesn't take much to be above average, but it does take a little bit more. And the reward for that ten percent addition is profound.

Summer

SINGING OUR SONG EVEN IF NO ONE IS LISTENING

Finding the unique song that we bring to the world not only brings us individual thrills and meaning. As the songs pierce the night sky, they can also move the few lucky enough to hear them.

I heard a birdsong pierce the summer evening sky as I was getting home one night. It was so stirring that I stopped what I was doing and scanned the area where the sound seemed to come from. I saw a small dot of color on a roof maybe twenty yards away. The bird wasn't spectacularly colored or endowed with any unique characteristics.

I held out my phone with an app that identifies birds by their songs and waiting with bated breath for the bird to sound again. It soon sang the same refrain as before, and the app identified it as coming from a song sparrow.

Sparrows aren't known for being flashy, overly vivacious, or exotic. In fact, in many novels, sparrows are used to signify the forgotten, the forlorn, or the barely scraping by. When the New Testament references the fall of a sparrow, it uses the bird to express the fact that God remembers the forgotten. Most of the time, we don't give sparrows much notice, fallen or otherwise.

Maybe the sparrow outside my house was singing because he was chemically induced to do so. Or perhaps instinct called him to let mates know he was around and willing to explore perpetuating his genetic code with a neighboring bird. But when I heard that passionate bird singing a hauntingly beautiful solo with no one other than maybe myself to notice, it made me wonder why he bothered.

But when I think of the lonely hunter from our distant past, who painted his mural in a cave that no one would applaud during his life, I get an inkling of why the song sparrow sings its song to no one but itself. In a world full of people urgently seeking attention and approval, it can be refreshing and restorative to do what brings us joy, not to gain the public eye, but because it holds meaning for us.

So paint that picture. Write that short story. Skip rather than walk. And sing your song because it helps you feel alive and present. Don't worry about how many likes you'll get on social media. Post it for you. What songs are inside of you that you can only sing for yourself? What song brings you such visceral joy that it would be nice to share with others but that you can enjoy alone as well?

Finding the unique song that we each bring to the world not only brings us individual meaning and joy, it can also move the few people lucky enough to hear it pierce the night sky as the song wells up inside of us and bubbles out with joy.

PROVIDING SHADE FOR FUTURE GENERATIONS

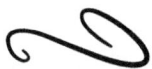

> It takes a special sort of kindness,
> humility, and sense of the common good
> to work hard on projects, knowing we
> won't be around to enjoy their fruits.

Have you ever walked through a city park with mature trees, lush lawns, and maybe a pond or water feature? I had some great city parks near my home, growing up, but I never really thought about who planned and designed, planted and cultivated, watered and nurtured these parks at their beginnings.

One afternoon in the late summer, I spent a good amount of time at Mt. Tabor, which is a gorgeous park on top of an extinct volcano in Portland, Oregon. The land for the park was acquired back in 1909—more than 113 years ago—and took several years to layout and landscape.

The person who had the vision for what the park could become and laid out the plans never lived long enough to see that vision completely realized. In the case of Mt. Tabor, there are certainly trees older than 113 years, so when the park was designed, those trees were incorporated into the plan. But hundreds more needed to be planted. Shaded picnic areas that are so pleasant on a hot summer day would not have been shaded when the designer laid things out. Beautiful groves of mature trees that nearly took my breath away, could only have been seen in the designer's mind's eye because, planted at the starting phase, those groves wouldn't have been nearly as impressive as they are today.

I realized as I walked along one of the well-used trails that cuts underneath the towering trees, that I often focus on short-term goals and possible achievements. Losing a pound or two. Writing a novel. Traveling to Europe. These are all worthwhile endeavors. But it takes a different kind of lens to think about the projects and goals and visions we can set for our families and communities, people and things that will undoubtedly outlive us and grow beyond our lifetimes.

So why work on such projects when we won't benefit from the end results? Sitting under such majestic trees reminded me of gazing up through the stained-glass windows of so many European cathedrals. The foresight that it took to plant the saplings that grew to create the shady park I enjoyed at Mt. Tabor is the same kind of generous foresight that built those cathedrals. So many of the day laborers who built those cathedrals never lived to see their completion, but they had other motivations.

Maybe a mason focused extra attention on a stone statue or other details, knowing that the extra attention would make the structure a little more special for the generations of people who would see his work. Maybe a carpenter took a little more extra care establishing the cathedral's rafters so that the roof would be more secure. In essence: they focused where they could add their skills, and in small, unseen ways, they made the buildings stronger by doing their best collectively.

So much in life doesn't really have a completion date. Are we ever done with taking care of family? Do we get to set our health aside once we reach a certain age or a certain level of fitness? Once we complete school, do we get a pass on learning more? And we can't forget all the unintentional work life throws at us when dealing with heartbreak, disappointment, loss, and pain.

Most worthwhile things in life don't have a fixed completion date, but maybe that isn't a bad thing. Maybe we can take a lesson from the planners of Mt. Tabor and find joy in making our contributions as good as they can be. Maybe we can find fulfillment in our knowledge that things are a bit better for our having lived our lives.

BUILDING UPON THE SHOULDERS OF OTHER PEOPLE'S SANDCASTLES

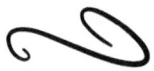

One of the hardest parts of legacy-building is detaching ourselves enough so that the next generation of sandcastle builders can build upon our foundations.

My sister and I set out to build a particularly sturdy sandcastle on the Oregon coast. It was one of those somewhat rare warm and sunny days on the Northwest coast, and so my sister and I prepared for quite the extensive operation. I would be the first to admit that I am no engineer. I'm not particularly mechanically inclined, and I was glad to move beyond the two required math classes in college. But it seemed to me that one way to protect the sandcastle against the changing tides was to dig out a very deep and fairly wide mote. My thinking was that when the waves rose with the night tides, they would slip into the mote and leave the structure of the castle intact.

Of course, there are many other variables, like how strong the foundation of the structure was and how quickly the waves rushed up against the mote, but we did our best. In the end, we had a mote that was almost as deep as I am tall. We included a few decorative flourishes to the castle, but with all the time and attention we gave to the mote, we didn't have a lot of extra attention to give to the castle's structure. By the end of our efforts, we were both pleased with ourselves, and excited to see if anything was left the next morning (though we both expected there to be no evidence of our efforts the next day).

To our delight, when we visited the beach the next morning, the castle was still standing and, in fact, about half of the mote was still there too. We congratulated ourselves on building something that could withstand those sometimes-rough tides, but we really didn't have any interest in building the castle back to its original glory. Instead, we spent time flying a kite and reading in the sun.

Then I spotted a mother and her daughter (who appeared to be maybe three or four) walking along the beach, picking up sea shells. The little girl seemed very focused on gathering the shells and collecting them into her shirt tails that she used as a makeshift basket. But then she spotted the sandcastle.

While keeping close tabs on her shells, she ran the best she could to the sandcastle. I still remember her delightful laugh when she saw it. I wondered what she would do next. Would she destroy it? There is something satisfying in totally demolishing a sandcastle, so I wouldn't have blamed her if the thought crossed her mind. But, no, what she did next has been a lesson for me ever since. She crouched down and carefully placed several of her shells into the moist sand of the castle. She thoughtfully chose which shell would fit best on the turrets and used a stick to dig out some of the mote. The mother and daughter worked on beautifying the castle for about a half hour—an amazing amount of time for a child that young to stay focused and dedicated to such careful work.

By the time the pair left the castle, it had been transformed into an ornate and repaired work of art. Something that my sister and I had built and left behind had taken on a life of its own, completely independent of our efforts or supervision.

I doubt the little girl remembers that particular experience. Maybe her mother does though. Either way, when I think about the little added enjoyment the mother and daughter might have experienced because my sister and I built something that they found worth adding to and enhancing, I get excited.

What kinds of legacies are we leaving? So often I find myself clinging to my own self-importance, as if that sandcastle could only continue to exist with me to watch over it. One of the hardest parts of legacy-building is sharing the vision and purpose and need behind what matters to us in a way that others will feel inspired and excited to pick up our flag and carry on. In most cases, to do this effectively, we have to detach ourselves enough that the next generation of sandcastle builders can make the castle their own.

Every situation calls for a different approach but I've thought about a few general steps that can help us celebrate the act of passing the torch to others.

- PREPARE IN ADVANCE. If we have enough time to thoroughly enjoy building our sandcastle, we are much less likely to feel cheated when we see others enjoying what we leave behind.

- BE PRESENT. Sometimes we feel resentment when others delight in changes to things that have mattered to us in the past. Important family traditions might change over time. We leave jobs where we've put our heart and soul into projects only to see them shift significantly when someone replaces us. But by fully engaging in what we are currently doing and by really sucking out the marrow of each experience, we can feel certain that we have made our contribution and be more comfortable leaving space for others to make theirs.

- **SHIFT THE PICTURE OF WHAT SUCCESS LOOKS LIKE.** If we set the goal of commanding our sandcastles as long and as fiercely as possible, then any change or invasion from others will be seen as a violation. We'd naturally protest if that were our objective in building sandcastles. However, if the goal is to enjoy the experience of building them and hoping it makes it through the rough tides, we can accept and even exult in seeing others build on what we leave behind.

So let's build our sandcastles. Dig our motes as deep as we can, and revel in the thrill of seeing others add beautiful additions to our legacy.

TAKING CARE OF OURSELVES SETS US UP TO ASSIST OTHERS

We need to be taking good care of ourselves—sleeping, eating, taking time for our own recharging. We can't draw from a dry well.

Summertime always makes me move into emergency management mode. Not so much because I deal with a lot of daily crises in my own life, but since I work for the U.S. Forest Service in a wildfire prone area, I have to relearn the lingo and get used to more daily briefings on the daily operations and evacuations. This focus on emergency management often reminds me of an experience I had that has similar underlying life lessons.

I took swimming lessons as a kid, but my technique was sloppy at best, so when my mom offered me the chance to take swimming lessons again with my younger brother, I took advantage of the opportunity.

> **Swimming is tough. I admire anybody who is proficient at it. At certain points in my life, I've thought it might be fun to compete in triathlons, and though I think I could do the running and biking effectively, the swimming deters me every time.**

I did my best during the lessons, and one of the final segments in the course was connected to water safety and water rescue. The instructor told us that saving someone who is drowning is much more difficult than the movies would have us believe. If the person drowning is panicking, they can drag the rescuer down with them, and if they are unconscious then the rescuer has to be able to swim carrying his or her own weight as well as the weight of the person being transported. That's why tossing a lifeline to the victim, rather than swimming out to them, is preferred.

Using this experience, we learn the importance of a few things:

- We should know our limits and our qualifications.

- If we're not the strongest swimmers, rather than jumping in after a drowning person, toss in a lifeline.

- Be willing to let go of ownership so that the greater, underlying purpose can be achieved.

- If the goal is to save a drowning person, maybe we don't need to play the typical hero, striding into deep water to save them. We should use the safest and easiest method to achieve that goal.

We all celebrate the miraculous rescues that heroic individuals perform all over the world, and we should honor and respect their sacrifices. But just like my swimming instructor's wise admonition said, if we swim out to rescue someone who is drowning, we might make the rescue effort more difficult for trained emergency crews. Especially if both we and the person we are trying to rescue end up needing help. Let's put on our own flotation devices first, then try to do so for others.

BECOMING THE SHADE ON A HOT DAY

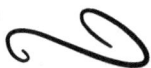

We could become the shade for those struggling under the heat of stress, disappointment, or fear.

One morning in early August, I was sitting out on my balcony enjoying some breakfast and some quiet reflection as I watched the sunrise. I know a lot of people love sunny, hot days, but there's a reason I live in the Pacific Northwest rather than in Miami or Phoenix. I don't deal well with a lot of heat or direct sunlight. I guess I'm kind of like my hydrangea bushes that I had as company that morning.

After sitting outside for a little while, the sun was beginning to be a bit bothersome, and I debated whether I should try to embrace it or go inside. But something shaded me from the sunlight. At first, I thought it was a cloud, but when I looked up, I saw that it was my young apple tree that I have growing in a big pot in the corner of the balcony. The leaves were filtering out the sunlight so that I could easily tolerate it for quite a bit longer.

I was surprised by the gratitude I felt for that tree. I bought it as a bare-root, dormant plant in the spring. For those who haven't planted a bare-root tree, let me tell you, they don't look great. Mine was a single stick, a few feet tall, with a few scraggly branches and some dangling roots. No leaves whatsoever.

It is quite the act of faith to keep watering a pot with nothing but a stick protruding out of soil.

But around early June, the stick started to show some very small, delicate leaves. Soon after, leaf clusters gave way to new branches, and a few months later, that stick transformed into something very much resembling the classic apple tree with healthy leaves growing on many thriving branches.

To grow from that stick that I received from the nursery into the verdant tree that I enjoyed that morning, the tree had to work rather hard. It had to start manufacturing chlorophyl as soon as the first leaves sprung up to energize other growth. It had to expand its roots so as to capitalize on the water I provided it. And it had to maintain its trunk, healthy and strong enough to withstand some decent wind gusts, although the stake and tie I attached to it helps some, I'm sure.

And because of all the effort that my tree put into developing those dark green, healthy leaves, as I sat there, I thoroughly enjoyed the shade it provided from the progressive heat of that morning.

Wouldn't it be amazing if we could become the shade for those struggling under the heat of stress, disappointment, or fear? I think most of us would love to help and support the people around us and especially the people we love and care about. But just like my apple tree needed to put in some time and effort before it could be a source of shade for me in a literal sense, we need to take some steps to grow so that we can provide relief for others who we see struggling. We can focus on developing nourishing habits that will help us to metaphorically put down stronger roots and healthier leaves that can then build helpful, self-perpetuating cycles that will lead to a greater capacity for us to help others.

And to be that shelter would certainly bolster the one enjoying the shade, but it would also bring rich experiences to the one providing that shade. The tree gets energized by growing leaves that take in the sun, and in a similar way, we can take in motivating energy from being aware of and willing to assist with the challenges others face. Through our willingness, we increase our growth and learn to ask sincerely and completely, without judgment or condescension, if they would like help, and then, having the necessary reserves of time and energy to actually provide that shade, we can help cool the sunburns that life gives to us all.

POTENTIAL IS A LOT LIKE A BOX OF ACORNS

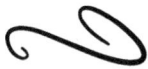

We never know how much of a difference helping one individual might bring to this world.

I was assigned to be the parking-lot monitor at my church's annual summer barbecue. The job didn't require much more than wandering around the parking lot so no car break-ins would take place. I was grateful for the shade that some large oak trees provided throughout the lot. And after making a couple of rounds, I made a discovery.

The ground surrounding the oak trees was littered with acorns of various shapes and sizes. Some were green, which means they had probably been blown down in the last major wind storm, while others were rich earthy-brown tones. I also noticed that, to large extent, where the acorns landed when they fell determined whether or not an acorn would remain intact and potentially capable of sprouting, given the right care.

The acorns I found in the soil had been, by and large, either opened and gnawed on by animals or had started to decompose in the rich and wet soil that Western Oregon is famous for. And most of the acorns that had fallen in the parking lot stalls or well-driven paths had been smashed by cars. But I did find a lot of viable acorns in the gutters and near trash cans, and rather than let them get smashed, I collected several dozen to take home to plant.

While driving home from the barbecue, I couldn't help but think about how similar people can be to those acorns. It's sad to admit that I too-often disregard the people I walk past on the street or drive past on the road. And maybe that's a saving grace. We only have so much attention available to give, and if all of it was caught up in getting to know or showing care to millions of complete strangers, we wouldn't have any time left to focus on the people we do know and love.

I might not be the right person to nurture and "plant" everybody I meet. (In this analogy, *planting* means to mentor and nurture and care about, not the other cultural definitions the word can imply.) Most people wouldn't accept help from a total stranger, even when offered. But we could all collectively care for and nurture some of the people we meet and with whom we interact. If we all did that, all of the acorns would be taken care of. None would rot away, be smashed under tires, or forgotten near trash cans.

What a different world we would live in if we all paid just a bit more attention to the people on the fringes of our lives and cultivated those relationships a bit more so that none of them were lost. We would certainly discover many vibrant relationships if we chose to nurture relationships with those on the fringes of society who might feel broken or forgotten.

Just like an oak tree has the potential to send out acorns that could grow into hundreds of thousands of new seedlings, we have the potential to make a difference by helping those around us. And there is no telling how much joy and positivity one individual might bring to this world. Moreover, we have no way of knowing which acorn will grow or what small act of kindness might strengthen someone who is struggling. But we might be exactly the right person in the right situation to nurture that individual into the sunlight. And what a remarkable experience that can be.

MEETING PEOPLE WHERE THEY ARE

We can't entirely remove obstacles and hardships from off people's backs, but we can make it a little easier, and that bit of difference, can make all the difference.

Fifteen years or so ago, I often had the notion to hike certain mountains or trails, and if the mood hit me just right, I would drop everything and go.

I've worked for the U.S. Forest Service long enough that I've wised up. Nowadays, I always tell someone where I'm going and when I should be back.

I haven't been in too many dangerous situations, but on that particular day, I was hiking Mount Ogden. The mountain poses a significant challenge. It's about sixteen miles round-trip, and it's a pretty arduous uphill climb: eight miles uphill most of the way. On top of that, the last few miles are a straight scramble across loose rocks and gravel that zap energy fast.

I started the hike on a summer day around noon, thinking I'd be back by five or so where daylight is available quite late into the evening. But because the trail was so arduous, it took me longer to get up to the top. My hiking boots didn't fit right either, so I developed horrible blisters all along the bottoms of my feet. I was wincing with every step and telling myself, "Okay, just got to tough this out. Put one foot in front of the other."

I was preparing to take every step of the way back to my car alone. I couldn't count on anybody else knowing where I was or when I should be back. And after about three or four miles of the downhill track, my feet were really, really hurting. And it was getting dark. And I was rather miserable. Though, I wasn't hypothermic or seriously injured, and I was still confident I'd make it down.

But then I heard a voice calling, "Chris?! Chris?!"

Relief flooded over me, and I nearly broke down and sobbed right there in the middle of the trail. My sister was five or six switchbacks below me—two miles away from the trailhead. I didn't ask anybody to hike up. I didn't have a cell phone at the time. Most people didn't back then. No one that I knew of was watching for my return. It wasn't until later that I discovered, that a few days before, my sister had overheard me talking to a friend about my plans to hike Mt. Ogden. When I didn't show up at home after dark, she and my mom decided to head up the trail to see if they could find me. With the late time, they worried and had hiked up the trail to meet me.

I still had to walk down the mountain that day, and I had to travel those two miles on my horrible feet. But the experience of having two people to cheer me on and to take some of the weight off my feet by taking my pack and giving me their shoulders to lean on, made all the difference. Those two miles were so much easier, so much more doable, because I had help. And then when I got back to the house, my mom and sister were kind enough to help bandage my feet and disinfect the blisters. (Though my feet hurt for weeks.)

There's a balance that we need to pay attention to when helping those who are struggling down the trail. First, we need to figure out what trail they might be on and where they might be along that path. When we find them, we can't carry them—not when they are miles from the trailhead—but we can carry their backpacks and give them a shoulder to lean on. We can cheer them on and match their pace so they don't feel pressured to go faster than they are able to go. My mom and sister did this. They met me on the trail and walked with me at my pace, but they didn't let me stop. They met me where I was and offered just enough support to keep me going.

It's one thing to meet people where we are, but it's something different when we meet them where *they* are. There is such a need for people willing to share in other's challenges without taking the learning opportunities away—a need for determined people who are willing to help others make solid steps forward at the right pace.

It might look something like helping a family member who is struggling financially develop a budget, but not giving them money. It might look like attending meetings with a friend who is dealing with an addiction (when invited) and being there for them when cravings creep into their life. Or it might look like providing a listening ear and empathy for someone who is dealing with depression or another mental illness.

This could translate into caring about how others experience the world and looking for ways to remove small obstacles and stumbling blocks, rocks and pebbles that they might stumble over along the trail—maybe offering your shoulder to lean on—without trying to take the steps for them.

I've got to think that that support would be as significant for the people in your life as it was when my mom and sister showed up on the trail for me. Maybe someone comes to mind that you could reach out to right now. Maybe you can make their day just a little bit better, just a little more doable. We can't entirely remove obstacles and hardships from off people's backs, but we can make it a little easier, and that bit of difference, can make all the difference.

CLEAN OUT THAT WATERING CAN

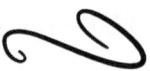

*Let's clear the leaf and dirt litter from
our lives so that our lives can flow
more freely and authentically.*

In the midsummer, there always comes a day when the wet Oregon spring gives way to full-on summer. And when that transition happens, I have to remind myself to start watering the plants on my balcony. It's a wonderful thing to know that, for months on end, if I leave on a week-long trip, my outdoor plants will be fine until around the drier summer season.

So, as I like to do with the start of new seasons, when I reached the midsummer of 2022, I made the process of watering my plants into a bit of a ceremony. I dumped out the wet mixture of leaves and dirt and old spider webs that had accumulated inside the watering can during the winter and then washed and dried the outside. Then I filled the large can to the brim and commenced the inaugural watering session of summer.

I live in a four-story condominium complex in an urban center, so all of my outdoor plants are on a large balcony, which one might think too small to hold so many plants. But after a decade of living in my place the number of plants out there has become quite substantial. I also have some new fairly large fruit trees in big pots that I'm growing from bare root starts, and so I have to make sure they get good drinks.

After refilling the watering can a second time and just before filling it for the third and final time, something dawned on me. I had been so focused on the visible parts of the watering can that I totally overlooked the nozzle. Soon after I started watering with the first load of water, I'd noticed that there wasn't much water pressure, and when the water dwindled to a trickle, I automatically thought I needed to refill the can. So I did.

But, before filling the can for its final use, and upon further examination of the funnel that leads to the nozzle, I discovered leaves and dirt debris blocking part of the nozzle. Not only did it prevent the water from pouring out as freely as it should have, but it also meant there was water left over that I wasn't using. In fact, each time I replenished the can, there were several ounces of water left over.

Just like the watering can, we each have leaf and dirt litter in our lives that keep us from fully embracing new opportunities or hold us back from fully enjoying some enriching experiences.

Do you have some habits you have yet to commit to changing? Are time-management quagmires sucking up your time and energy without paying back a residual return on your investment? Are there relationships that you know should be cut or that you should dedicate more time and effort toward?

Once we are honest enough with ourselves to admit that we can use some adjustments and some *nozzle cleaning*, the difference will be immediately felt and seen—just like I saw with the last refill of water that I poured on my eager plants. Once that leaf and dirt litter was gone, there was nothing to keep the water from flowing freely.

IT'S A GRAND OLE COMPLICATED FLAG

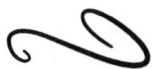

We don't have to think, look, or feel the same or eat the same foods or speak the same language or love or worship the same way. But we should try our best to make our country better by caring for those around us and using our time and muscle for good causes.

Flag day is a day set aside to commemorate the act of the fledgling congress that established the original design of the United States national flag. "The Union be thirteen stars, white in a blue field, representing a new Constellation."[3] Woodrow Wilson made the day a nationally recognized day 139 years after that act of Congress back in 1916.[4] But why do we mark a day for a flag? We have plenty of other holidays that commemorate the founding of our nation, significant figures in our nation's history, and days to draw our remembrance. What value does this particular holiday, which commemorates a rectangular piece of fabric, hold in any practical sense?

Did you know that until the motion was made to designate one unified flag, there were numerous flags flown over the battlefields of the Revolutionary War? Since a lot of the battles were fought by militias organized by regional or even ultra-local leaders, many groups had their own banner to rally behind. Although each militia and regiment held the same goals and aspirations as they confronted the formidable British military forces, without one banner to gather around, each soldier fought their own battle rather than fighting a unified battle as part of an army with a central cause.

That central and unified flag was a symbol of a greater principle: a unified nation. There is something beautiful in believing in things larger than ourselves, whether that be human goodness, nature, God, the force of science, family, or country. But that beauty is enhanced when we think about the concept of loyalty that is parallel to the principles that the United States was founded upon but that is sometimes misunderstood.

Patriotism is an inherently messy concept. Political parties claim to be more patriotic than the others, people attempt to show national pride by flying the American flag in their car windows (or stuck to their bumpers) and in their front yards. Some people even claim that nationalism is the same thing as patriotism.

Of course, in its most basic form, patriotism represents a desire for an organization—whether it be a family or a nation—to be better. Coupled with that is a level of commitment to contribute to that betterment.

National news and politics grab our attention because local newspapers and news stations are dwindling and iconic national news anchors thrive by using attention-grabbing tactics. But when push comes to shove, much of what we can do to make our communities (and ultimately our country as a whole) better happens through small and simple acts of service. Helping out at our local elementary school, serving on a city committee, volunteering as the chair of our neighborhood association, organizing food drives, or cleaning up our neighborhood park.

These kinds of patriotic actions might not be flashy. They might not be life or death like the actions taken by those who rallied around that original flag more than 245 years ago. But they can represent the same ideals that spurred the concept of one central flag for the soldiers to rally around. We don't have to think, look, feel the same or eat the same foods or speak the same language or love or worship the same way. But we should try our best to make our country better by caring for those around us and using our time and muscle for good causes—let's celebrate that.

CHANGING THE WORLD ONE MOMENT OF GENEROSITY AT A TIME

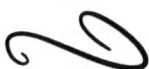

We all need help from each other, so by sharing our generosity in a unified cause for good, we can, in a real sense, change the world for better.

One of the most remarkable stories of heroism that I've ever heard is about the Thai soccer team that was rescued from a network of caves back in 2018. Sometimes, we think of heroes as the people we read about or watch thrilling movies about instead of the people walking among us. But this story rekindled my belief in everyday heroes.

The soccer team was composed of young teenage boys who visited a cave after their soccer training. They went a few miles into the complex underground network of caverns, but unbeknownst to them, at the surface far above them, early monsoon rains had started to flood the cave.

Before the boys knew what was going on, their way out had been flooded and it was impossible for them to walk or swim back to safety. But that's when the truly magical part took place. Through the coordination of local and international engineers, thousands of volunteers, and a few brilliant, world-renown cave divers, a successful rescue was planned and carried out. Not a single boy was lost.

Nothing of the sort had ever been undertaken. The rescue plan called for the cave divers to reach the boys after swimming several miles through the flooded tunnels, then to sedate each boy one at a time, and have a cave diver guide the sedated boy, geared up in scuba gear, back to the entrance of the cave.[5]

That event captivated the worldwide news media for several weeks. And it pulled in thousands of volunteers from around the world. There were crews brought in from the United States, Europe, several Asian countries, and Australia. It brought the world together in a neat way.

One of the Thai leaders, talked about what it took to safely accomplish that monumental task of rescuing all twelve of the soccer players and their coach when no one thought it was possible. He said it was based on two fundamental concepts: generosity and unified effort.

I've never heard that concept described in a more beautiful way. We often talk about working for the common good, but that doesn't quite encapsulate this concept. The added element of generosity that drives that common good opens the door to for us to work together in spite of our differences. There were definite differences among the countries involved in this rescue, but they still rallied around this cause and rescued these thirteen trapped people from the cave.

How easy is it to let a person's political view cloud our view of the whole person? Before we are even aware it has happened, we've made too many unfounded and unfair assumptions. Sadder still, is when we assume to know what kind of a people those around us are based on scanty inputs. It shuts down cooperative learning and communication and that miraculous unified effort that is only possible if we lean into our curiosity about people.

What will be our unified effort today? We're probably not going to be involved in an underwater cave rescue. But what cause will drive our generosity enough to join forces with those who may be different than us in order to accomplish something we couldn't do alone? It may be as simple as donating some food to a food bank. Or maybe it's reaching out to visit a friend we haven't talked to in a while who might view the world differently than we do.

We all have needs. We could all use a warm smile or hello from a friend. Everyone could benefit from a visit. It's remarkable to think of what kind of influence for good we could be if we combined our individual acts of kindness and generosity and let them rippled out into the world.

FORGED IN THE FIRES OF FRIENDSHIP & KINDNESS

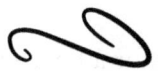

When individuals have to flee their homes because a wildfire threatens them, we reconnect with our foundational human need for community.

Recently, my agency prepared for a major wind storm that could have made the wildfires we were already dealing with much larger. The wind also had the ability to make new fires flare up. After so many summers in a wildfire adapted ecosystem, this was not a new phenomenon for me, But since 2019, we've had particularly severe fire seasons. I've had a hard time not looking back on those desperately long, sad, and hard weeks when hundreds of thousands of acres of Forest Service land were burned.

But I've had to remind myself of the acts of heroism—big and small—that I've witnessed and chronicled as a digital storyteller. And when I think of the dozens and dozens of examples of selfless service that I've seen and of my chance to see communities rally behind firefighters and celebrate in the safety and small victories that some communities have experienced, my faith in humanity—to do remarkable things and rise from the ashes of the darkest moments—is brought to a bright flame.

One night, a resident in a small, close-knit community was woken by a firefighter pounding on her door, giving her a chance to get out of the path of an approaching wildfire. The community member credited the firefighter for saving her life, and I had the wonderful job of connecting the community member with the firefighter who had done her vital work so humbly that the community member didn't even know her name.

I also gathered materials for a heart-warming story about a forest law-enforcement officer who found a baby owl in the path of a wildfire. Its parents were nowhere to be found. So what did the officer do? She put the baby owl in a Yeti cooler and delivered it to a bird sanctuary. Other folks offered their homes as temporary shelters during evacuation orders. During evacuations, community meals were also provided free of charge, with warm smiles and handshakes all around.

Sometimes, it can seem as if our species has forgotten that the only way we've ever been successful has been by working together. But these stories of connection remind us that none of us can make it on our own. Whether or not we pride ourselves on our independence, when individuals have to flee their homes because a wildfire threatens them, we reconnect with our foundational human need for community. Our challenge as citizens of a modern world is to find a way to choose that sense of common good that connects us with others and can grow inside of us. One that can motivate us to look outward and value others a step above our immediate self-interests because we recognize that there is something more worthwhile in togetherness.

It's amazing to watch people step up in remarkable ways when a crisis springs up. We understandably herald people who sacrifice and work hard for the good of families and communities. But that same sense of togetherness, knit through a web of thousands of threads of goodwill, common good, and community strength, is also important when the forest isn't on fire. In fact, in order to build a community that we can rely on, we need to build lasting relationships when things are calm and safe. That way when emergencies arise, we'll have built automatic habits of caring.

WISDOM OF SHEEPDOGS

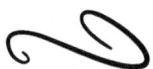

Just as sheep dogs protect and keep sheep safe by guiding them along the path, listening to mentors, wise friends, and family can set us on a safer path.

Each Labor Day, for the last two decades, my family and I have visited the Soldier Hollow Classic—an event where sheep dogs try to herd sheep around an obstacle course of sorts. The dogs are absolutely amazing! When I say that the dogs drive the sheep through an obstacle course, I am not talking about an air-conditioned arena with barriers that block certain routes. These dogs herd the sheep about a quarter mile up steep hillsides, then downhill a quarter mile, then back up halfway. As they do this, they cut across the field through a couple of barriers. The sheep are then separated as the dog and handler work together to move the herd, grouping those with collars and those without. If the handler—the owner of the dog—has enough time and skill, he attempts to drive the sheep into a small pen while the dog creates a wall of pressure to keep the sheep from bolting. Each element helps the human–dog team to accumulate points. The goal is to drive the sheep as calmly and as straight as possible across an invisible line that angles across the field.

The fact that a single dog can drive sixteen sheep in ninety-plus degree weather, running several miles throughout the course, absolutely boggles the mind. There have been times when the dogs have penned the sheep at the end, and after working so hard, were totally exhausted.

Of course, this contest is a game of sorts. But the skills that the dogs exhibit are vital to their everyday working lives where they herd animals on farms for their handlers' livelihoods. The dogs keep sheep and cows together and drive them according to the needs of the handlers. The dogs also provide protection and, through the directions of their handler, are aware of dangers and challenges that the sheep or cows are totally oblivious to.

Of course, to the sheep or cows, the dogs pose a simple threat. Some of the sheep seem less afraid and more annoyed by the dogs, but in either case, the dogs are seen as an obstacle to the sheep's liberty and freedom to wander the field and eat as they go along as they please.

Freedom to choose our own destinies and paths in life is a wonderful thing that we should all enjoy. However, like the sheep and cattle, it's healthy and helpful to have boundaries set and to follow the guidance of the people we trust rather than doing what we want, whenever we want to do it.

I was an independent kid growing up, and I'm sure I drove my parents absolutely crazy because, like sheep, I had the tendency to wander off and explore, whether we were camping, hiking, or at a mall. I wandered everywhere. I was quite certain that I knew what I was doing and where I was going and why, so it never made that much sense to me that I should stick with my family or that my exploration needed boundaries. I was certain I could find my way back. However, when I was five or six, that independence got me into some trouble.

We had taken a fairly extensive hike up a canyon in the Salt Lake area, and on the way back, I was tired of hiking at the rate that the rest of my family had adopted, so without clear permission, I ran down the trail, thinking that there would only be one trail and I would meet my family at the trailhead. Little did I know that there were multiple forks in the trail. I happened to take the wrong one. I reached the bottom of the trail by cutting off-trail, and instead of exiting to the trailhead parking lot, I exited directly to the road. I didn't know what to do next. I could have walked either direction for a while. Eventually, I probably would have run into the trailhead. I was certain the trailhead was off that particular road, but at the time, I wasn't certain whether the best option was to use that trial-and-error method or to stay put. I felt very much like the sheep that get alarmed quickly but don't always know what to do next. Thankfully, I recalled seeing a Woodsy Owl sign near the trailhead on the drive up to the hike, and I had come off the trail right underneath that sign. So that's where I sat and waited.

As you can imagine, my mom was rather alarmed when she got back to the trailhead and I wasn't there. So much in fact, that she called search and rescue. A helicopter was even activated in the search. I was unaware of any of that activity and felt quite safe and secure where I was. Though I clearly wasn't in a position to find my own way either. Eventually, a member of the search and rescue team found me, and I discovered that I was only a few hundred yards away from the trailhead parking lot. I reconnected with my family just fine. This story has a happy ending, for me at least, although my mom had a stressful hour or two.

Sometimes in life, parameters are for our good. Had I followed the rules about not getting too far ahead and staying on the trail that my mom had set for me, I doubt I would have had my unfortunate adventure. And although we can seek freedom and total flexibility, having some boundaries can be good for us. They show us what is possible and help us enjoy healthier relationships and to find ways to avoid pitfalls that could be much more dangerous than sitting under a Woodsy Owl sign. Just as the sheep dogs protect and keep the sheep safe by guiding them along the path and reminding them of the perimeters in which they can be safe, listening to mentors, wise friends, and family can set us on a safer path.

RUNNING TOWARD THE MORNING SUN

Just as we choose to enjoy the bright sun as it shines upon us, each of us can choose how we see the experiences in our lives.

I try to go running most mornings. It gives me a good reason to get out of bed before the day becomes warm and offers me a chance to do something good for my body as I run around my neighborhood, which has a unique flavor. So there was no surprise when I hit the pavement one particular summer morning, like I had hundreds of times before.

I typically run a large square that loops me back to my house. In the summer months, since I live in the northern stretches of the U.S., most of the path is shaded by great trees and city buildings. But as I near the final stretches of my route, there's a section where I run facing directly into the sun.

Most of the time when this happens, I squint and try to shield my eyes. I feel the heat beating against my face, my eyes strain, and my steps are heavier and a bit uncertain as I push through that blinding sunlight. Then, once I can duck under a building's shadow again, I'm quite happy.

But on one particular day, I took a different approach. I chose to look at the sunlight, not as an annoyance, but as a blessing. I tried to imagine how welcoming a bright sunny morning would be to someone who had been stuck inside their house—maybe because they were sick. I tapped into how it felt to be a kid on a summer morning that was absolutely bursting with potential. I honed in on the sensations brought by bright warmth and light and color that I experienced in the moment. And seeing the sun in that way brought on a thrilling sensation that lightened my feet and added an extra bounce to every stride I took. I even started smiling as my eyes squinted with the bright sunshine.

I can't say that I was thrilled by that blinding light, but that changed vantage point shifted those moments dramatically. Instead of gritting my teeth and squinting in frustration, I was able to lean toward that brilliant sunlight and recognize the goodness it brings.

Just as we choose to enjoy the bright sun as it shines upon us, each of us can choose how we see the experiences in our lives. We can grit our teeth and simply endure in the hopes of future moments when we will better enjoy life, or, with a fullness of hope, we can tap into the goodness of the moments we are already living.

THAT DOG-EAT-DOG WORLD SHOULD JUST TAKE A BREATH

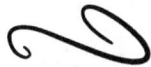

Sometimes it can be healthy to care a little less about where we are headed and just enjoy the ride.

I was driving down a lonely stretch of highway when an SUV pulled up beside me at a traffic light. There wasn't anything remarkable about the SUV as far as I could tell, but then I took another quick look at what was in the back seat. A dog had its nose sticking out the window with its eyes closed.

That dog was a picture of complete joy and contentment in the present, and as I thought about it further down the road, after parting ways, I asked myself, *Why wouldn't that dog be near heaven in such a situation?* He had cool wind brushing through his fur, warm sun beaming down on his face, and he was presumably riding along with a family who loved and cared for him. Even more, he was taking in new sights and sounds and smells that he could explore and use to expand his horizons.

Wouldn't it be nice if more of our time was spent in a similar fashion to how that dog experienced that ride? I'll admit that I spend a lot of my time worrying about what's happening next or stressing about problems that have risen in the present or wishing for different outcomes in any number of arenas. What would it take to enjoy a nice moment completely and single-mindedly?

As I see it, we would have to:

- Recognize that things are all right—as long as we are breathing, not in serious pain or in a life-threatening situation. In fact, if we don't find ourselves in one of those situations, then most things are rather good.

- Give up everything that isn't occurring in that very moment so we can focus on the pleasure of the present.

- Close our eyes and let sensations wash over us. (Maybe we don't need to close our eyes like my dog friend did, but sometimes doing so helps shut out the distractions so we can focus on our other senses.)

- Care a bit less about where we're going and focus on where we are right now.

It's true that life is short and precious. So we should suck the very marrow out of life experiences, but in a paradoxical way. This path doesn't include a hurried or stressful rush from one experience to the next. Often the best way to truly experience life is to focus on the goodness that is around us right then, just like that dog in the car lived in the moment, not caring where they were going, he just enjoyed the ride.

Fall

THE POWER OF ONE TOUCH IN OUR LIVES

It's amazing how much of an accumulative impact one person can make in our lives.

Soon after my initial brain injury, lots of things had to work together for me to become a regular, functional kid again. A lot of that had to do with physical therapy and other physical needs, but I also lost about half a school year of learning, and I had the added challenge of figuring out how to learn with an almost-but-not-entirely different brain. Academics had been so easy for me that I had never really learned how to work hard on concepts like reading, writing, or math. So it was a hard realization that, if I wanted to be successful in school again, I'd have to relearn somethings that weren't so easy for me anymore. One of the biggest obstacles at the time was reading.

Learning how to read again was such a weird experience. My right brain was completely healthy. Once I was able to sound out the letters that made up words, I quickly grasped the concepts. But that took training. And I was a pretty lazy kid back then.

Enter Sophie Richards.

Sophie was my next-door neighbor when I was a kid. I had my quirks and rough edges, like most kids do. I'm sure she had qualms about me, but she also had a magical way of grand-mothering all the kids who knew her. And her way of grand-mothering was exactly the kind of support I needed.

Sophie invited me over to her home to read with her each weekday morning before school, which must have made our meeting time around 7:00 a.m. By this time in her life, she had traveled all around the world, and her study, where we'd read in the mornings, showed it. She had chessboards from Turkey and wooden figurines from Kenya. To be honest, being invited to such a cool room was enough for me to get up a half hour early to practice reading with her.

Kids pick up the fact that some people are respected because of who they are and what they've done in the community. And though I didn't have the words to describe my feelings back then, being in Sophie's home, full of amazing souvenirs from her world travels, I knew that Sophie was someone worthy of respect. And I didn't want to disappoint her. With Sophie, I tried harder than I would have on my own or with a speech therapist. Beyond that respect, though, Sophie gave me just the right kind of motivation—she was patient when I struggled to sound out words, and she never let me get away with skipping one. She paid such close attention, and I felt like—although she had her own life and her own family and aspirations—when she was with me, I was the most important thing in her life.

As I reflect back on this period in my life, typing these words that come so easily to me now, while sitting in my study, which is full of books that I love—even if my study isn't nearly as cool as Sophie's—I can't help but think about how my life today could be quite different if Sophie hadn't reminded me that I enjoyed reading—at least once I got past the hard work of translating words into ideas.

We only met for a year after my hospital stay. Had I not met with Sophie, would I have gone to college? Probably. But would I have pursued a master's degree? Would I be working in a profession that requires constant reading and writing? I don't know. But very likely not.

So often we aren't even conscious of the true impact supportive roles, such as Sophie's, make in our lives. Consider not only tutors, like my dear friend, but also school janitors who make an effort to smile and exchange warm-hearted jokes. The crossing guards, who not only keep us (and our children) safe while crossing the street, but also make us feel ready for the school day because we know in our hearts that at least one person really cares about us. The neighbors who know how to balance healthy boundaries and privacy, but who would do just about anything, at a moments' notice, to help us if we were hurting or in a bad situation.

Oh, how grateful I am for people like Sophie Richards, who provided just the right kind of support and encouragement and hard love that has led me to who I am today.

THREE CHEERS FOR TEACHERS

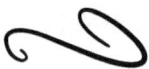

> We can't say that we deserved or have earned the kind of teachers who made our lives exquisitely richer. We can only be so grateful to have happened upon them and to have had their powerful influence shared with us.

One recent fall evening, I had the great joy of meeting up for dinner with a dear old high school teacher, Margaret Rostkowski. Ms. Rostkowski had a tremendous impact on me, and I remember now what a profound difference teachers make in the lives of their students. Teachers change lives. And Ms. Rostkowski changed mine in very important ways. She taught English, Mythology, and Creative Writing, and she was also the advisor for the high school writing journal. I think I took every course she taught, although it was never my intention to focus on English in college.

Beyond her excellence in teaching, she was even more impactful because of the way she treated every student who entered her classroom—with the dignity and high expectations that every student longs for, even though they might not always enjoy the amount of effort living up to such expectations requires.

> Isn't it interesting that those teachers who demand
> the most of us quite often are also our favorites?
> I don't think that's a coincidence at all.

Those high expectations teach us that we are capable of more than we sometimes believe and that we are worth the attention.

Margaret Rostkowski's high school classes were run like college classes. She never accepted late work. She held us accountable for reading assignments, but not with gotcha pop quizzes. Instead, she spent the next class discussing the reading with the assumption that we were prepared. Maybe some of her students didn't respond as powerfully to that approach as I did, but by allowing me the opportunity to take full responsibility for my education, I understood that I couldn't shirk my duty to be prepared for class.

In her classes, Ms. Rostkowski brought attention to some precious details that I grew to expect even though none of my other classes offered such unique elements. I remember so many early mornings when the sun would first peek over the eastern hills. I'd walk into Creative Writing, fill a mug with herbal tea and hot water that somehow was always at the ready, find a seat with an inspiring view of the mountain range outside the lead-framed windows, and see her wrapped up in one of her fantastic shawls, smiling at me with her curious and intelligent eyes and inviting me to lean into the challenge and wonder of learning.

The amazing thing about these remarkable teachers is that they continue their important work despite the fact that so few students have the words or the emotional and social maturity to recognize and verbalize their thanks. And to think that these teachers are already asked to run metaphorical marathons without shoes, water breaks, or sufficient training time. And they keep at it for decades, nurturing fresh crops of students year after year, with a keen curiosity of how each year will play out, hoping that a few students will truly embrace the material that means so much to them.

I'm so incredibly grateful to have stayed in contact with this dear, dear teacher so that I can appreciate and celebrate her amazing efforts after the fact, at least. Even though it's now been a couple of decades since I last took a class from her, that night, at dinner, she showed me that her commitment to, interest in, and excitement for my success and continued discoveries remained. She asked about my writing of course, but she also celebrated in my world views and challenged me in others, using her diplomatic but direct way that I've always loved.

While I was with her, I viewed learning as a journey and a thrill and not only as something that I had to do to graduate.

We don't meet very many teachers quite like that. Teachers endure such long days, absorb so much of their children's painful life stories, seek to inspire children who often are not interested in what their teachers are trying to teach, and all of this while getting paid a meager salary under sometimes very rough conditions. I hope everyone has at least one teacher like Margaret Rostkowski. We can't say that we deserved or have earned the kind of teachers who made our lives exquisitely richer. We can only be grateful to have happened upon them and to have had their powerful influence shared with us.

PUDDLE HOPPING AND OTHER THRILLING PROSPECTS

We can all use more puddle-hopping, jungle-gym-climbing, fall-leaf-leaping, and tree-climbing. If we were to feel more encouraged and comfortable doing these sorts of things, we'd enjoy a richer perspective, just as we would get a different perspective sitting high up on a tree branch than we would from the ground.

During a lunchtime walk, I had just rounded a corner when a girl with her mother walked past me, heading the other direction. The girl seemed awfully excited, and I assumed she was going to dance class because of the studio straight ahead of them. Then I noticed her wings and her unicorn horn and her bright-pink rain boots. I beamed a completely genuine and spontaneous smile at both of them. I fought the urge to laugh out loud from pure delight at seeing the girl being exactly who and what she wanted to be.

I complimented her on her very stylish wings, and the girl said thank you in the sweetest way. Her mom had been guiding, half-nudging her in the right direction, and after smiling back at me, she continued her trajectory toward the front door of the studio's building.

But then the girl stopped.

Right in front of her was a deliciously glassy and huge puddle just begging to be tromped in. Her mom immediately picked up on the girl's thinking, and in an attempt to cut it off at the pass, explained that they didn't have time to enjoy the puddle and that her boots would get all wet, which was totally reasonable and sensible.

I watched for long enough to see the girl make a couple of quick splashes around the rim of the puddle before heading into the building. I was glad that she got a chance to dabble into the puddle.

Why don't we relish in the sheer joy of jumping into puddles? Especially as adults? Why is it that we so rarely put down the guise of appropriateness and enjoy the thrill of simple and messy and fun things?

For one, our footwear is rarely designed for it. I'll admit, I'm kind of a shoe fiend. I don't buy shoes very often, but I take good care of them, and I tend to look for bargains on high-quality shoes so that they last a long time. Because of this, many of the shoes I wear just aren't designed for puddle-hopping. In other words, if I want to be a bit more comfortable taking the leap, so to speak, into enjoying messy but thrilling experiences, I am better off wearing rain boots than leather loafers. Sadly, sometimes I find myself wearing nice shoes because I'm afraid that if I don't, the people around me will think less of me—think me less intelligent, less professional, or less good at what I do—instead of recognizing my encouragement of others to jump into the creative and rejuvenating world that we lived in as kids, where joy was more spontaneous.

It's an interesting phenomenon, adulting. A lot of the steps we take to become what we call an *adult* are good and healthy. Learning how to be a bit more responsible, punctual, conscientious, and healthy are all fabulous goals. But, somehow, we also learn, through cultural observations, that adults should choose the least messy route. Which, in lots of contexts, can be beneficial. The task, then, is to decide what messes are worth cleaning up. Getting some paint on grubby clothes might be worth it. It could be worth it to take off our shoes by the side of a river and let the mud ooze through our toes. And yes, especially if we are wearing proper footwear, it can absolutely be worth it to get our feet a bit wet from puddle-hopping.

Still, sometimes as we go along the process of becoming adults, we have to convince ourselves that it's a good thing to forgo childlike activities for the sake of being responsible. And if we tell ourselves this enough times, we might get to a place where we aren't only willing to accept it, but we actually start believing that *responsible* is the only proper way of thinking. When we step up to our puddle, do we talk ourselves out of jumping because we're not dressed for it or we're heading to work and need to look presentable? Do we disregard that dream job because another one seems more practical? Do we put off learning to paint, or rock climb, or write, or play an instrument in part because we know we won't be immediately proficient and we fear that our attempt won't be good enough? Do we avoid the puddle outright because we are certain that puddle-hopping is wrong? Not just messy but wrong?

The world is in dire need of more unadulterated joy. We can all use more puddle-hopping, jungle-gym-climbing, fall-leaf-leaping, and tree-climbing. If we felt more encouraged and comfortable doing such things, we'd enjoy a richer perspective, just as we would get a different perspective sitting high up on a tree branch than we would from the ground. Not to say that one perspective is necessarily better than the other, but that we need both to triangulate our path in life forward. So the next time you wake up on a rainy day, pull on your rain boots and slicker and hop in a puddle or two. It could do us each a world of good.

THE GRAND ADVENTURE OF IMAGINING WHO WE WANT TO BE

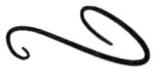

If we aren't one hundred percent satisfied with the person we are today, we don't need to despair. We are all works in progress—characters in our own make-believe game—trying to determine who we want to be.

I distinctly remember the day I first met Audrey, a bright and inquisitive third grader who joined the after-school program organized by the Salvation Army in Bloomington, Indiana. I didn't know much about her background, other than the fact that she and the other kids in this particular program typically came from rougher family situations and that Audrey seemed to have a harder time warming up to people than the other kids did. But when she did warm up to people, she went all out.

That first day, I found her playing with Pokémon figures, making up grand adventures for them, all by herself in a corner in a large classroom while the other kids played noisily around her. I sat down on the carpet next to her and asked her the names of the characters. She outlined the dozen or so character names, a little about each back story, and their individual superpowers.

Before long, Audrey allowed me to enter her imaginary world where a particular flying Pokémon character had to continuously save the others from their terrible fates. Somehow or other, the flying character saved the day every time. I was particularly excited when I was given the great honor of playing the flying hero. Audrey coached me on the proper way to lead the story, based on her far more superior knowledge of that character as well as the other Pokémon characters.

This make-believe activity filled a couple of hours until it was time for Audrey to go home. But on the subsequent days, Audrey insisted, to my delight, that we continue where we left off the day before. Over the following weeks, we played out dozens of dynamic adventures, ranging from cliff dives to underwater sagas, to cloud kingdom rescues and beyond. Our conversations never veered too far from the game at hand, and we were both okay with that.

It was amazing how liberating and recharging it was to be fully immersed in a different world, becoming a new character with powers new and fantastical.

I ended my volunteer experience at the Salvation Army a couple of months later as I graduated with my master's and moved to Oregon. Audrey and I exchanged handwritten notes for a couple of months, but without that face time and make-believe play to connect us, eventually, I stopped hearing back from her.

A decade later, the surprising power of imagination has stuck with me. I believe that we never really lose our imagination, but I also believe that if we don't give it the attention it deserves, it can go dormant and we can forget that it's there. Why is it that as kids we can uninhibitedly jump into new worlds and assume new characters, but as adults we struggle to decide who we are, let alone have fun playing rolls beyond our own?

But maybe that pursuit of our unique identity is actually interwoven into those role-playing games the kids play. Perhaps those imaginary games are important not only for the sake of creativity, but also to offer the kids a chance to take on different roles. To metaphorically shed their skin and try on someone else's attributes for a short-term run to determine how it fits. Child psychologists have found compelling evidence to back this up.

Philosophers throughout the ages have posed questions about what personal identity means and what it consists of, as well as its origins. But in my life experience, none of us are destined to fit into one pre-packaged personality or persona construct. Rather, we get to reinvent ourselves as we go along, basing our personalities on the interactions we have with others, the disappointments and triumphs we experience, and the values we discover to be of worth to us as individuals. This means that if we aren't one hundred percent satisfied with the person that we are today, we don't need to despair. We are all works in progress—characters in our own make-believe game, trying to determine who we want to be.

SHOWING OUR TRUE COLORS

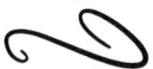

Let those rich reds, yellows, and oranges shimmer with the brilliance of knowing who we are and why we do what we do.

Think back to those wonderful elementary school science lessons when we learned things like what makes a lightning strike and what causes the seasons. A lesson that I thought about recently, as I sat out on my balcony taking in a beautiful fall sunrise over Mt. Hood, was focused on what makes leaves change color.

I absolutely love seeing the brilliant yellows, oranges, and reds that pop up all over my neighborhood in the fall. But what makes these gorgeous colors? In reality, the leaves have the pigment inside them all the time. It is just overshadowed by the chlorophyl-rich nutrient-gathering organelles that make the leaves green. In the fall, trees naturally stop gathering the energy from the sun that they use during the spring and summer to grow branches, height, and fruits or seeds for propagation, and instead prepare for winter.

Isn't that a beautiful metaphor for how we often hide our true and brilliant colors behind the guise of staying busy, productive, and useful?

We rush from one task to another, stretching every time-management trick we know to fill our days with work or kids' activities or church responsibilities or tidying up. And if we're not careful, we can start to believe that doing those things makes us who we are instead of being firm in who we are first and letting the things we do personify us.

I'm definitely not against filling our days with activity and projects and work. That's the nature of modern life, and being engaged in good causes with good people can be incredibly rewarding and meaningful. But there's a key added element that transforms a busy life into a meaning-rich life.

It's a subtle but important distinction. In some ways, it flips those activities on their heads, and when we live beyond being busy and productive, to the point of certainty in who we are and what matters to us, our activities are motivated by our deep sense of self. We no longer rush around, hoping that by filling our days with good activities, the universe will magically reveal what our purpose and meaning in life should be.

There's really no shortcut to figuring out who we are and what we care about. My personal journey with self-discovery took me through an exploration of experiences that were emotionally charged. In essence, the best and worst experiences of my life. In digging through these experiences, I was able to parse out why they were so impactful. I realized that providing support, hope, and gentle nudges for people in my life who are discouraged is a driving force for me and what I'm meant to do on this planet. By using those stories again, I was able to pull out my core values—empowerment, worthwhile work, mastery, and clarity. We all have a unique purpose, drive, and reason for being on this earth, which means we all have unique contributions that only we can provide.

So let your true colors shine through those busy activities. Let those rich reds, yellows, and oranges shimmer with the brilliance of knowing who you are and why you do what you do. That way, when you are faced with the prospect of adding another activity, all you have to do is decide if it aligns with who you are and what you value most.

IF A TREE CHANGES COLOR IN THE WOODS, DO WE NOTICE?

There are very few things more beautiful than a tree lit up by its fall splendor. But the tree doesn't do it to look better or be noticed.

I've got to admit that I love the feeling of checking things off my to-do list. At the end of the day, if I don't catch myself, I'll think back on all the things I accomplished and measure the success of the day based on how many tasks I completed (or how well I accomplished the tasks). I'll get innately frustrated with myself if I don't knock out at least some tasks.

I'd imagine a lot of us are similar in that way. And there's nothing wrong with using a to-do list to ensure our time is prioritized so as to maximize our efforts on the things that matter most. But sometimes to-do lists become the master rather than a tool to be used by the master—which should be us. I reflected on that while I was… well… drawing up my to-do list for the day.

My office has a window that looks out to the street. The street is lined with good-sized maple trees, and at the time, the leaves on those trees were just starting to turn to their fiery burnt-orange hue. While looking at the leaves sway slightly in the breeze, I had a thought: *I wonder if trees use any kind of to-do list.* I chuckled at imagining a tree with a satisfied smile on its trunk as it crossed off items like *seal up holes for better insulation, begin process of color change with task completed by mid-October, begin dropping leaves by November 1...*

Natural processes might follow certain timelines and predictable patterns, but they are certainly not ruled by checking things off a list. Trees' successes aren't measured by how many tasks they knock out on any given day. Instead, they use their days soaking in as much energy as they can, growing as many leaves as they can in order to maximize that energy absorption so that they can be best prepared for winter. And here's the *ah-ha* moment for me: the trees do it whether or not anybody notices or praises them. And the evening after a major wind storm when the skies were gray and the trees lost a lot of those precious energy-producing leaves, the trees don't dismay over unfinished tasks.

Perhaps a part of why trees have evolved to be so stable is because they live much longer than we do. We strive to be more and accomplish more, to be better looking, smarter, healthier, better informed, and important in the eyes of others. But there's something we can learn from the trees' approach...

There are very few things more beautiful than a tree lit up by its fall splendor. But the tree doesn't do it to look better or get more notice. The tree makes that transition to prepare for what's coming. The tree has an internal motivation all its own that just happens to mean that we get to enjoy beautiful fall colors. Maybe that's a lesson we can learn from fall trees—a successful day might look quite different than how we normally see it. Rather than feeling like a failure if we don't cross every item off our to-do list, we can reflect back on the rich moments of the day, be grateful for the people who were kind to us, and celebrate the moments we were kind ourselves.

WHAT HAPPENS AFTER THE CAR CRASH

It is easy to shift blame or justify our mistakes, but to build true character, we must act the way we profess to believe and cheer for those around us to do the same.

While returning home after a speaking engagement for my church, I was unfortunately hit by another driver who rolled out of a parking lot without looking or stopping for oncoming traffic. The driver sped off, and I wasn't able to get the description or license plate number of the car. Thankfully, my car is older and not worth that much, so I sanded down the scrapes left by the other car and touched up the paint myself. It took a bit of time and effort, but it wasn't that big of a deal, and I'm thankful no one was hurt.

After the incident, as I drove the few miles home, I was initially shaken and frustrated. I thought of the annoyance and inconvenience of getting my car fixed and the possible embarrassment of driving around with a scraped-up car while I waited to take it to be fixed.

But then, thankfully, I was able to shift my mindset. It dawned on me that neither I nor the other driver was hurt, that my car was still drivable, that no pedestrians were involved, and that, after some introspection, I didn't really harbor any ill will toward the other motorist. In fact, I was surprised to realize that my overarching emotions were sadness for the other driver and curiosity as to why he or she would have hit me and then driven away.

I don't know what the other driver's situation might have been. Maybe kids were in the back seat, distracting the driver, or maybe the driver was preoccupied by troubles that I had no clue about. But whatever the reason, doing the wrong thing (by not stopping and exchanging insurance information) will inevitably lead to less desirable outcomes for the other driver.

Recognizing that we have made a mistake can be one of the most challenging things we do. So much so, that sometimes we try to hide from the responsibility of our mistakes or try to pawn the blame off on someone or something else. We are all wonderful at playing the justification game—projecting our circumstances away from our own actions and decisions.

But contrary to the anxiety and fear that mistakes can bring, in the overwhelming majority of situations, people appreciate it when we recognize our mistakes and do our best to make recompense. And though that recompense might mean some hard things and some hard moments down the road, often, the side-effects of this acknowledgement heal relationships so that they are even stronger than before. On top of that, we are able to add another data point to our overarching geotagged map of lived experiences. Like a rewarding and intricate geocached treasure, by collecting datapoints on our path toward greater understanding and empathy, a more detailed map starts to appear. And that map reveals to us, and to those around us, our true character.

One concrete way that I've found to reveal my own character is to reflect on what I stand for and what that projects into the world. Am I honest with myself first and then when interacting with others? Do

I believe good principles strongly enough, and have them engrained into my mindset enough, that I live according to those beliefs, even when—perhaps especially when—it would be more convenient to do otherwise?

That is one of the greatest sources of hope that I have for humanity—believing that though people might not always live up to their ideals, most of us still have at least the aspiration of living up to them. And that is why I've eventually been able to let go of the frustration of having my car damaged without being compensated. Because I know that I don't always measure up either.

If we can juxtapose the two ideas—the hope for a just and character-driven world on one hand and ways to improve ourselves on the other—we'll be able to forgive ourselves and others, while still holding ourselves and our communities accountable for trying to be a bit better than before.

REPLACING OUR TIRES TO AVOID THE WRECK

Once we've gotten through the initial struggle that is inherent with change, we can find excitement in the possibilities posed by that change in our life.

In preparation for a business trip, I dropped off my old, reliable Infiniti at the shop to make sure it was safe for me to take on a couple-hundred-mile stretch. The auto shop reported back that my tires were completely bald and that they absolutely did not recommend driving it anywhere, let alone on a two-hundred-mile road trip. I can take a hint that blatant. I purchased four very nice new tires that should last me several more years, given how little I drive.

We often believe that certain things will stay in good working order and fail to plan for their eventual repair or replacement. It's so easy to wait and cling to our hopes that we'll escape yet another trip without a flat tire. That we can go without seeing a dentist or delay that physical exam or rely on caffeine to tide us over after several weeks of mediocre sleep.

But life has a way of catching up with us, doesn't it? A car wreck can be disastrous and cost much more than a vehicle's value, not to mention the cost of stress and possible bodily injury. Much more than new tires or other minor repairs. If we don't take good care of our dental hygiene, we'll end up with a root canal, which costs a lot more than a regular dental visit or cleaning. A major operation can cost exceptionally more than a regular check-up. And that extra hour of sleep each night can keep us safe and mentally sharp so that we can be worth more to our business or employer; it also might keep us from dangerously dozing off at the wheel.

As humans, we naturally feel a strong pull to keeping things as they are. Psychologists call it the status quo trap. We're pulled in the direction of the status quo for a few reasons.

Deciding that we need to take an alternative path might force us to admit responsibility, like with our example of avoiding a visit to the doctor or dentist. The status quo is comfortable because the alternative would make us face the reality that maybe we haven't been taking splendid care of ourselves.

Taking a path other than the status quo probably requires a bit of work—like with my tire replacement task—it's easier to ignore the need for new tires and continue to drive on the old ones because taking the car into the shop takes time and money.

So how do we break away from the status quo trap so that we can face the consequences of not doing what we should to help ourselves be healthier, well-rested, and more energetic, all while saving our teeth? I've found that following these three steps makes a difference:

- Stop exaggerating the annoyance or cost of getting things done.

- Recognize the cost-growth that comes with each delay. (The threat of a major expense grows if we put off regular upkeep.)

- Incrementally set aside time or small amounts of money in preparedness for unexpected expenses.

I still struggle with the status quo trap, but when we recognize and understand the problem, it makes it harder to ignore. And in some ways, it can be exciting to take the long-view approach instead of living from one disaster to the next.

EMBRACING THE RAINSTORMS WITH A GOOD PAIR OF RAIN BOOTS

Wearing shorts and flip-flops will not make the December weather magically change, but we can learn to love wearing sweaters and jackets and rain boots with pizazz.

I typically start my morning by scrolling through my New York Times and weather apps. One morning in early fall, I was thrilled by what I saw. Not because of anything particularly positive. Goodness knows that positive news is a rare treat these days. No, I was thrilled because the weather forecast said there was a thirty-seven-percent chance of rain and that it would only reach the mid-seventies.

Come January, I imagine I'd have a similar reaction for the opposite reason. After a couple of months of rainy days and cloudy skies and jacket-wearing temperatures, I'm usually ready for a sunny day.

Early fall carries other reasons to be excited about cooler, wetter weather as well. Every rain storm is a blessing. It means communities that have been hard hit by devastating wildfires (several in recent years, many of which have dealt with evacuations and lost homes) will be able to breathe a collective sigh of relief and the beloved landscapes can start the remarkable process of regrowth and renewal. The air can become more breathable. And trails, once again, hike-able.

But what is it that makes me excited for the change from hot, sunny days to cooler, wetter weather in the fall and then long for dry, warmer weather in winter? It probably comes down to seeing the positive side of change. It's such an overused statement that change is hard. That statement lacks nuance.

Sometimes we long for change. Sometimes change can't come soon enough. Sometimes change is an answer to prayers and hopes. Other times, change doesn't come when we most desperately hope for it. Think about a family member dealing with a debilitating illness. We long for a change, but sometimes it doesn't come. So how can we look forward to change as well as the lack of change?

I guess that's one of the life lessons we all need to strive to learn—to be willing to accept what may come and love it just the same. But we can also take certain steps in this direction:

- Focus on the good that comes into our life, whether that be a rainstorm when we need rain or we are faced with a hot stretch.

- Recognize that there are multiple perspectives to everything. A rainstorm could be a godsend to a farmer and trigger a fallback plan for a wedding planner.

- Try to make the situation as positive as possible, even when the outcome cannot be controlled. Wearing shorts and flip-flops will not make December weather magically change, but we can learn to love wearing sweaters or jackets.

MOMENTS OF JOY

Change is a major influence in our lives, and often we don't have much say about the changes that occur. But sometimes we can celebrate the sunbreaks after days of cloudy skies or thoroughly relish the cooler weather after weeks of hot days. And by focusing our attention on those simple pleasures, we can look forward to the positives, whatever they may be, through many more times and seasons.

LETTING OUR MISTAKES FLOW DOWN RIVER

People are resilient and, most of the time, very eager to forgive. Let's be easy forgivers of ourselves too.

I recently dug into the origins and meanings and traditional practices of Rosh Hashanah, and though I am definitely not a Jewish scholar, there was a particular practice that appealed to me. The practice is called Tashlikh. The practice calls for the recitation of prayers and the casting of our sins and misdeeds into flowing water, either in thought or through the symbolic use of bread crumbles or pebbles.

When we think about sins, we too often think about our shortcomings. The times we snap at our children or pound on our steering wheels in traffic or think ill of our neighbors or coworkers. Sometimes, we think about the things we should be doing more of or better or with greater gusto. In either case, the concept of repenting for those misdeeds inevitably implies a negative connotation. No wonder we don't like to think about self-improvement when we are looking at things through those lenses.

But the concept of Tashlikh is about letting go of old ways. It's meant to be a liberation from the weight our regrets put on us. Certainly, if we have hurt others, then part of evolving beyond those issues is making amends, but much of our psychological and emotional baggage is self-made, isn't it? We know how to do better, and since we never fully achieve what is ultimately possible, there's always room to feel bad about our performance day after day.

So let's cast our regrets and self-criticism and the weight of actions we think we should have taken or should have done better into the river. Let's celebrate the fact that every day gives us a chance to try again and that people are resilient and, most of the time, eager to forgive. Let's be easy forgivers of ourselves too.

Forgiving ourselves is often more difficult than forgiving those who have hurt us. We know the thoughts that motivate our actions, and sometimes those thoughts are not pleasant or kind. But I'm grateful that we can cultivate the ability to make good decisions with some consideration of what happens next. Feelings of doubt, discouragement, and disappointment can be powerful, but if we start with small acts that change our perception of ourselves, we can cast those doubts and misgivings into the river and watch them roll downstream.

Think of the reasons self-doubt talk is wrong. Come up with the reasons you are strong and capable right now. Then cast your doubts and misgivings into the waters to be carried away.

WHAT THE WORLD NEEDS NOW - EMPATHY

When we find a way to survive and move forward through hard times, those challenges are transformed into incredible gifts for others.

If I could point a finger at a single attribute that our world could use more of right now, it would be empathy. Empathy is the remarkable ability to not only feel sorry for others, to not only hope things work out for them, but (in some real sense) to feel the pain others feel. This shared experience can create a much deeper connection and bring comfort in a way few things can.

A while back, I had the opportunity to speak to a church congregation about how we can still hope for good things to come during our hardest times. In that address, I relayed my experience of waking up in the hospital and not being able to walk or talk, then going through years of therapy to regain the skills that we typically take for granted.

After the meeting, a wonderful older gentleman pulled me aside and told me how much he appreciated my talk. His granddaughter had recently had a brain injury similar to mine, and she was relearning how to walk and talk and was using a wheelchair. Instantly, I felt a deep connection to this genuine and warm man, and though I had never met his granddaughter, I felt a connection to her as well.

I didn't have a morsel of profound insight to give this good man, but I think when we can empathize with other's challenges, the connection matters a lot more than tips or pointers. When we feel terribly alone in difficult circumstances, it can be overwhelming. We can't see where or when or how those challenges will or can ever end. But when we connect with someone who has walked similar paths to our own and made it through to the other side, we recognize that we can survive our current circumstances too.

Understandably, few of us seek life challenges. Goodness knows, challenges find us frequently enough. But when we do face hard things, we are given a gift that we can share with others. And once we've shared that gift of common connection and understanding, the gift we've given is bestowed back on us through the love we feel, the stronger relationships we enjoy, and the gratitude we feel for our fellow human beings.

Challenges test us, and sometimes in the direst circumstances, they bring us to our very limits. But when we find a way to survive and move forward through those hard times, those challenges are transformed into incredible gifts for others. They give us the chance to fill the shoes others will walk in.

CELEBRATING AND HONORING THE COURAGE & SERVICE OF VETERANS

Many of the simple kindnesses that we experience daily come off as so commonplace that we don't recognize their miraculous nature.

I was out running my regular few-mile route around my neighborhood, as I do most days, when I ran past a couple of distinguished-looking gentleman with snow-white hair cropped nicely around veteran baseball caps as they walked toward the veterans memorial near my home. I go past the memorial so frequently that I am ashamed to say that I haven't always given it the gravity it deserves. It's been a long time since the United States has been inserted into a major conflict where enough of its citizens have been involved for us to fully realize the horrors of war and the singular courage that service-people exhibit.

I can't begin to grasp the magnitude of the sacrifice and willing service these two gentlemen who I ran past must have given to protect and defend our country. And hundreds of thousands more have served faithfully since the discontinuation of the draft. It was a serious reminder that I need to show greater respect and honor to those willing to die to protect me, my family, and my community.

The term *courage* has lost some of its original depth. It takes some strength of character to do anything hard, whether that be speaking up for those who are marginalized, trying to lose a few pounds, or being our true selves with our friends and family. But it takes a different kind of courage to face an enemy that is set on killing you and still follow the order to advance and rescue fallen comrades.

As I ran past the two men at the veterans memorial, I thought about my ancestors, many of whom served in the military and fought in wars, never expecting anything special in return. "It was my duty to serve my country" is all they say about their service.

The concept of acting out of a sense of duty sometimes gets a negative connotation. These days, we are told to find our passions and be true to our sense of self. Yet, there are some things much bigger than any one of us. There are ideas worthy of sacrifice. We absolutely owe veterans more than we can give. But gratitude is a good first step. Maybe the next step will be looking for ways to emulate their dedication by supporting causes that work for the greater good.

MODERN-DAY GOOD SAMARITANS

If we set a rule that commits us to help anybody we see who is hurt or in need of help, we'll have the necessary mindset to step in when a situation arises.

One recent fall morning, I did what I do every few days: I took some recycling and trash down to my condo's garbage facility. I was dreading it because I knew what I would find when I got there.

The facility technically has a key-code entry to restrict access to only residents, but there's enough space above its walls and fence for someone to toss in trash and other materials—like mattresses and broken furniture. And although the waste management company takes care of the refuse inside the trash and recycling containers, they don't go out of their way to clean up around them.

You can guess how my trip to the facility played out. Little by little, the trash and discarded items had accumulated until I opened the locked door. I was absolutely disgusted. One can turn a blind eye to a little bit of trash—justify not feeling responsible for cleaning an area designed to house trash—but this was embarrassing.

For a few seconds, I weighed my options. I could do one of three things:

- Complain to the building management and shove the responsibility on them

- Rationalize leaving it alone since I wasn't personally responsible for the mess (Besides, what would cleaning it up teach the people responsible?)

- Clean it up, knowing that I would feel better about the situation and that it would make taking out the trash a nicer experience for my neighbors

I chose the last option.

To be completely honest, it felt great to be a part of the solution—for the first five minutes or so. After that, I gritted my teeth until it was reasonably clean. So far, the area has remained clean, although I'm not certain how long that'll last.

This experience reminded me of a psychological phenomenon called the *bystander effect*. The bystander effect refers to a predictable occurrence where people in public places or common areas assume that someone else will do the prosocial thing. Basically, help or clean up. The problem with that line of thinking though, is that everybody else thinks the same thing. Even though everybody would benefit, at least a bit, from someone stepping up and doing the right thing, often no one does.

The classic example of this comes from one of my favorite studies. In 1973, researchers observed theology students as they were presented with an opportunity to do the right thing.[6] In this scenario, the students were told that a major exam would take place in a different building on the other side of campus. The experimental variable—the thing that was varied among groups—was the amount of time the students had to get across campus. Some students had plenty of time, others had barely enough if they hurried, and one group was told they were late.

What the students didn't realize was that along their path the researcher had staged an actor lying on the ground and in obvious distress. How many students do you think stopped to help?

When I've heard this study described in classes, and when the results are talked about, the emphasis is always on the huge majority of students who didn't take the time to help. Roughly two-thirds of the students never stopped. The interesting thing is that the percentage of those who helped varied widely, depending on how hurried the students were. Among the low-hurry group, over sixty percent offered help. In the medium-hurry group about forty-five percent stopped, and only ten percent offered assistance among the extreme-hurry group. Ironically, the subject the students were focusing on—that took them from one building to another—was the parable of the Good Samaritan.

There have been many other famous experiments geared around the same theme as the bystander effect. And two questions seem to impact our decision to step up and assist:

- Is the situation clear, and do I know what's going on?

- Am I in a hurry?

The beautiful thing about our knowledge of the bystander effect, though, is that we can break this human tendency. By knowing that people don't usually help, we can choose to do the right thing even when we're in a hurry or when things are ambiguous. If we set a rule that commits us to help anybody we see who is in need of our help, we'll have the necessary mindset to step in when a situation arises. We won't even have to weigh our options because the decision will already be made: we are one of the helpers in this world, and that's just what we do.

Winter

LET GO TO EMBRACE THE NEW

It might take some effort to head in a different direction, but if we do our homework and make the best decision we can, more than likely, we'll end up in a better situation that helps us move forward.

One chilly Saturday morning, I decided to replace a rhododendron that I'd had in a pot for several years. It had never flowered, but it had been leafy and healthy most of that time. It had also seen a dramatic decline for a couple of months before I made my decision.

I went through every excuse to hold on to it: *I've had it this long—I hate abandoning it now; maybe it'll turn around; it doesn't look THAT ugly with yellow, shriveled leaves.* But, ultimately, I took the plunge and said a quiet goodbye to what was left of the rhododendron and a thank you for the joy it had brought me over the years. Now the remnants of the plant are doing more for the earth in the compost pile.

This experience has made me realize how often I behave exactly the same way in regards to other aspects of my life. How often do I justify holding on to bad habits or waiting to start productive ones simply because I'm comfortable with that status quo? How long do I have to go to bed too late only to dash around in the mornings as I get ready for my first work meeting before I get to bed early and have a meaningful morning routine? Why do I buy into that false belief that I'm too busy to exercise *this* week but that I'll do better *next* week?

There is rarely a better time than now to start making positive changes in our lives. There are so many reasons why we don't start down a path that might lead to healthier decision-space, and habits. But in general, taking the first step is the only way to actually make changes.

There are many more consequential decisions that we make in life than to replace a plant. We choose our relationships, jobs, spiritual practices, health choices, clothes, vacation destinations, and our preferred brands, from cereal to toothpaste.

There is a huge library of resources out there to help us weigh the pros and cons of all of our choices. But once we have determined the best course, the path forward—away from what we already know—often requires a lot of energy and faith. It might even cause stress.

> **Now that I have taken the steps to replace my rhododendron, I have a lovely hydrangea that is doing incredibly well and brings me even more joy.**

It might take some effort to head in a different direction, but if we do our homework and make the best decision we can, more than likely, we'll end up in a better situation that helps us move forward. Then the magic of self-perpetuating goodness can kick in.

If we take small steps toward achieving our most important goals, even tiny steps, those small moves forward can snowball. For example, if I want to exercise in the mornings, I can set out my exercise clothes the night before and get up a little earlier, then take a walk around the block, I'm bound to feel some level of fulfillment. I'm likely to eat healthier. I'll feel better about myself, which means my interactions with coworkers and those with whom I come in contact will likely be a bit more productive and positive. By the end of the day, I'll have racked up several feel-good moments that I might not have had if I hadn't taken that walk around the block.

Everybody has their own keystone habit to start the ball rolling, but we all start on the path up a mountain at the same place—the trailhead. So let's take those first steps and be on our way.

DEATH BED GOAL SETTING

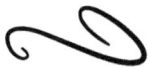

When we reach our death beds, who we have become will matter most, not what we have done or where we have been.

The book *Happiness of Pursuit* by Chris Guillebeau has been a great reminder to not lose sight of big ideas and audacious goals. It has been a reminder to strive to live the life I want and dream about, instead of embracing my comfort zone. If I had read the book fifteen years ago, I likely would have full-heartedly embraced it and felt validated. I was a goal-setting fiend back then. Case in point, when I was thirteen, I read John Locke's *Two Treatises of Government* and decided then and there that I would become the world's first international chancellor.

 I'm still goal-oriented. And I still have big dreams for myself. But I've come to realize that, while I set big goals, I also need to focus on each day as it comes rather than only calculating for the future. At thirteen, I was interested in striving for more and becoming more. Now I've filtered that against living each day as fully as I can.

Goals are inevitably future focused, and I still get caught up in the future tense. I've wanted to speak Spanish fluently for a long time. I've downloaded the apps and have had varying degrees of success with a study regime. If I ever want to really speak and understand the language, though, I'll need to dedicate time each day. Over a long enough period, I'd eventually accomplish the goal.

The reason I struggle to say more than "Where is the restroom?" in Spanish is not because the goal is wrong or because my desire to learn isn't strong enough. It's because I haven't made my goal into a disciplined daily practice. (I hope you will all hold me accountable to do better.)

There are all kinds of worthwhile goals, from micro daily goals to life-long aspirations. Throughout life, we can use similar techniques to progress toward all that we hope to accomplish. That way, when we're nearing the end of our lives, we'll have stories and memories rather than regrets.

Have you ever written a bucket list for yourself—things to do or experience before you die? Maybe one way of motivating myself to learn Spanish would be a four-month immersion program in Costa Rica. Then I could accomplish a large goal while checking off a bucket-list item. Spending time thinking about what experiences we hope to have in life is wonderful. If we don't articulate what we want, we are unlikely to stumble upon our desired outcome. At the same time, I don't see very many bucket lists that include "be kind to everyone I meet" or "spend more time listening" or "give friends my full attention when I'm talking with them." These sorts of aspirations aren't the kind that make great bucket lists, but they make wonderful daily aspirations. After all, when we reach our death beds, who we have become will matter most, not what we have done or where we have been.

I want to learn Spanish so that I can let native-Spanish speakers know that I value them and their cultural identity. I have a life-long aspiration to help migrant farm workers to live healthier and more fulfilled work lives. And those goals are geared toward me becoming a more useful and well-rounded person who can serve people in new ways. I'll be able to speak with and understand the needs of another group of people.

Of course, life rarely goes according to plan, even when we have the best intentions of helping others. Sometimes life throws serious curve balls at us. Debilitating illnesses happen when they are least expected, and they are never convenient. Relationships break down. Incomes come and go. Even our abilities can change in an instant. We shouldn't give up our dreams when serious setbacks hit us. If we have a strong enough sense of who we are and what we value, we can navigate toward rewarding aspirations, even if some of those aspirations need to change their shape and focus.

GATHER YE ROSEBUDS AND MAYBE STOP TO SMELL SOME TOO

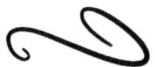

Might I suggest we take a lesson from the many world cultures that embrace the concept of having plenty of time because all we ever really have is *right now*. And now is an abundant resource.

Western societies have a certain way of looking at time. They tend to look at it as a very valuable, finite resource. Over the years, I've heard many varied sayings about time. On one hand, I hear how precious time is. On the other hand, I hear that we all have exactly the same amount of it—from the richest to the poorest people on Earth.

These concepts are meant to help us seize the day, so to speak—to take advantage of every moment as if we'll never get it back. It reminds me of that great scene from *Dead Poet's Society* when Robin Williams' character leads his class of awkward teenagers to the trophy room at the prep academy and whispers in their ears, "Gather ye rose buds while ye may… Seize the day, lads! Seize the day!"

Just reminding myself of that scene sends thrills down my spine. It's motivating, not only because Robin Williams' character is trying to help some troubled boys feel better in their own skin, but also because of the concept he is teaching. Namely, that time is so precious that we need to take full advantage of it and use it wisely.

Nearly all time-management programs and workshops and books are built around the same basic premise: how do we squeeze more out of our precious minutes and hours so that we can be more productive, feel more fulfilled, and do more? There is nothing inherently good or bad about this strategy. If people want to pack as much stuff as they can into a storage container, it makes great sense to pick up a trick or technique or two so that they can fit more into the same space and do it better than before.

Over the years, I've used paper Franklin Covey planners, original Palm Pilots, and old personal digital assistants (PDAs), and now I try to leverage my iPhone and desktop-scheduling apps to their fullest. And I have definitely embraced the doctrine of modern-time management. After opening my Franklin planner thousands of times over the decades, Benjamin Franklin's quote has been drilled into my brain.

> Doth thou love life? Then don't squander
> time for that's the stuff life is made of.
>
> ~Benjamin Franklin

But as much as we are immersed in the concept of time management, modern Western views of time are not the only way societies can or do look at this very precious resource. Psychologists talk in terms of two different time schemes. The kind I grew up with, complete with time-management devices and techniques and tight schedules and set timelines, is called monochronic time. Time is seen as a set chronology. It can be visualized as a timeline, and people with this sense take out blocks of time to fit in their days. The other way of looking at time is called polychronic time. In this sense, people draw out time as though they are drawing it out of a well. They drink up the amount of time it takes to live out certain experiences. In this way, there isn't a *right* length for a meeting to take. You're never really running late because what is being done in the present moment is important and meaningful, making it exactly where you need to be.

We can all see the strengths and drawbacks of these two senses of time. Countries with a monochronic time sense, like the United States, can achieve a lot. They can organize events, meetings, deadlines, flights, and product launches. Monochronic time has led, in part, to the United States' incredible productivity. I recently read that no country in the world works more hours on average than the people of the United States. But there are certainly drawbacks.

How often do we have a meaningful conversation with a friend or family member and feel a deep connection with relationship growth, only to have that disrupted by a nagging urge to move on to the next scheduled thing? There will always be something else we need to do, some task to perform, someone to see briefly, according to the predefined length of time.

Polychronic time alleviates that constant burden of being on time and filling our days with useful tasks and interactions. It replaces it with a pool of time that we can draw from in order to be fully present in the now. The trade-off is real though. Typically, countries that have a polychronic persuasion are less wealthy. In fact, as countries industrialize and transition into more developed nations, there are clear correlations between that advancement and a loss of polychronic thinking.

So what am I suggesting? That we should all abandon our schedules and timelines and iPhone calendars and go with the flow, enjoying the moment? Certainly not. Even if we could learn to see time that way, the nagging pull toward productivity and the reward of industrialism would be a constant driver for us.

What I am suggesting is that we enjoy some polychronic moments in our days, weeks, vacations, and work days. We can find time, even scheduling it into our day, if we need to, to just be. How remarkable would it be if we shut off the notifications on our phones and just enjoyed the connections at our next family get-together? How impactful would it be to carve out ten minutes from our day to cloud-gaze or enjoy something beautiful or to call up a friend and let the conversation go wherever it goes?

We all have the same 168 hours per week. Those hours are awfully valuable, no question. If we get to the point where our schedules become more important than the purpose and substance behind them, then might I suggest that we take a lesson from the many world cultures that embrace the concept of having plenty of time because all we ever really have is *right now*. And now is an abundant resource.

HAPPY BROWN HOG DAY!

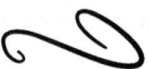

When we are curious, not only do we learn and experience more truth, but we also invite others to learn things with us.

When I was in preschool, my class had art, story, and nap time, although, back then, I didn't see the point in nap time, so my poor teacher put up with me using the nap time as more reading time. And I remember the day I discovered a neat new holiday. A large rodent-like creature who lives in the ground, comes up to the surface on February second each year, and if he sees his shadow that means six more weeks of winter. At the time, it was well beyond my cognitive abilities to understand why this rodent seeing his shadow and predicting more winter was an odd and confusing logic, but I loved the concept of the holiday—for one reason—it was new to me, which meant it was my job to make sure that everybody else new about it too. And that definitely included my teacher, Mrs. Porray.

So true to my quest to spread the word about this new holiday with a big rodent that has prophetic powers, the first thing I did when

I entered the classroom on February second was shout, with as much triumph as I could, "Happy Brown Hog Day, Mrs. Porray!"

Mrs. Porray was made out of rare stuff, I guess, because she smiled and tried to share in my excitement, but she was also a teacher and eager to teach me the proper name of the holiday.

"I think you must mean Groundhog Day, right Chris?"

To this day, I'm not quite certain why the concept of calling this new found holiday anything other than Brown Hog Day seemed so wrong to me. I remember justifying my reasoning. The animal was brown; therefore, it made more sense to call it a *brown hog* than a groundhog.

Given the fact that there were no groundhogs living in the wild in my part of the country, the creature might as well have been a mythical centaur for all I knew.

Most of all, though, I remember that I didn't like being corrected and that this triumphant discovery was turning into something much less pleasant than I had anticipated.

I went back and forth with Mrs. Porray until, with a wise smile and nod, she finally said that I could believe what I wanted to believe. Soon after this encounter, I realized my mistake, and now, as a fun connection between us, I try to send Mrs. Porray a note every February second, wishing her a happy Brown Hog Day.

What I've realized since discovering that the holiday is Groundhog Day, not Brown Hog Day, is that being inquisitive and open to other peoples' views of the world can be one of the most beautiful skills we can learn. When we are curious, not only do we learn and experience more truth, but we also invite others to learn things with us. That shared understanding can lead to richer relationships and wonderful discoveries.

When I think about my adult life, I have to admit that sometimes sticking to my guns, even though others have valid arguments that prove I am probably wrong, still holds a lot of appeal. So often, we like feeling right—that the world as we see it is in its proper order. It makes sense. As human beings, we have a strong need for assurance that we are safe and in control of our lives—both our now and our future.

These days, though, I try to be curious rather than defensive when people present information that I disagree with. Even if I am certain I'm right, there are always new perspectives that can add nuance to what I know. And being right, for me, rarely matters enough to damage relationships. I've learned a lot from Mrs. Porray's kind approach of gently correcting me about Brown Hog Day. There is so much I don't know or understand, and leaving room for correction opens the door much wider to gaining understanding.

JOY DURING THE RAINSTORMS

∽

When it's raining, we have a choice:
complain about getting wet or be excited
that trees are getting a drink.

One a rainy morning during my sixth-grade year, I was unusually early for my first class. Rainy days are rare where I grew up, and I was poorly prepared. My hair was drenched, as was my trumpet case. Since I was so early, the classroom was empty, other than Mrs. Wilde, one of the most impactful teachers of my life. She was sitting at her desk in the back corner and leaning slightly back, gazing at two rows of young evergreen trees that had been planted a year or two before.

As I set my things down at my table and did my best to dry off my things, I had the first tinges of a bad mood come over me. But then I turned to greet Mrs. Wilde.

At first, I didn't want to disturb her, in part, because I was in the middle of that awkward transition where teachers were rather intimidating and I was still eager to please them—Mrs. Wilde especially—but also because of the look in her eyes as she took in the serene scene outside her bank of windows. When she turned and saw me, she gave me a polite smile and nod. I smiled back.

"What are you looking at," I asked, instantly certain that that was the absolute stupidest question to have asked. Though, I didn't know what I should have asked instead.

She looked back at the trees. Beads of water glistened where they rested, tucked on branches and trunks. "Just watching the trees getting a drink," she replied.

I sensed that that was a profound statement; although, as I try to jump back into my twelve-year-old self, I'm afraid that the main thing that excited me was how I could use that phrase in a poem. Thank goodness, however, that I've had that experience tucked away in my memory banks to unpack many times over the years.

Out of that precious experience with Mrs. Wilde comes the thought that the physical experiences we face in life can be viewed as either good or bad things, depending on our perspective. Forest fires are terrifying, destructive, and deadly. They also renew soils and clear areas for new growth. Volcanic eruptions can destroy homes and ruin vacations to tropical paradise, but without eruptions, the islands wouldn't exist. Snow might mean a car crash to travelers, while, to fish, it might mean a stream in which to spawn and revitalize life. And yes, rain can be devastating for a bride with her heart set on an outdoor wedding. But, then again, it also provides a drink for those young pine trees.

Rain is absolutely nothing new in the Pacific Northwest. In fact, certain areas on the west side of the Cascade Mountains in Oregon can get nearly two hundred inches of rain per year. But rather than constant downpours, after short time living here, I'd grown to expect more of a gentle misting from November until late spring. Then came a day when the rain was torrential. Streets were so flooded that cars were stuck in pools of water with their engines submerged as they drove down residential streets. And I, unfortunately, had a meeting in downtown Portland that I needed to participate in. I took the train.

Portland has amazing transit, but we still have to walk from the train station to our end destinations, which in my case, was a few blocks away. I was prepared for that. I had my waterproof rain jacket on and had upgraded to a windproof umbrella. But almost instantly after getting off the train, my not-so-windproof-after-all umbrella was blown inside out with several of the wire components breaking off their hinges. Even my high-tech rain jacket was no match for the rain that blew at me from all directions.

In disgust, I tossed my broken umbrella in the nearest trash can, tightened the straps on my backpack, and steeled myself for the trek to the meeting location, prepared, yet again, for a bad mood to take over for the day. But then I thought about Mrs. Wilde and those young evergreens getting a drink. It wasn't an instantaneous shift, but gradually, a smile crept over my face and I imagined the happy evergreens in the Bull Run Watershed (a temperate rainforest that supplies most of the drinking water for the entire Portland Metro area) getting some wonderful drinks of water. And I thought about the wildfire that had burned through another portion of the same national forest the fall before. I thought about the strained faces of families who had been displaced by the wildfire as it headed toward their homes.

The rain didn't instantly become a joy, but the memory of Mrs. Wild's words made it a more bearable walk to the office. And by the end of the day and over the next couple of years, in true Northwestern fashion, I grew to appreciate those rainy winters because it meant the forests could stay green year-round.

When I go past my old middle school today, and when I see the towering trees that were once the same height as my sixth-grade self, I'm reminded about all the drinks of water those evergreens must have required to grow into the stately trees that provide so much beauty and shade for the school today. It's *so* hard to look at our hardships in any other frame of mind, isn't it? But the same rain that cancels a soccer game might have been fervently prayed for by the farmers who hope their crops will grow.

I am so grateful for Mrs. Wilde's wise thoughts then and on many other days since. I hope that future generations will catch a glimpse of the trees outside those windows getting a drink. Thinking of that seems a much healthier than complaining about getting wet.

WE CAN LEARN A LOT FROM THE TREES

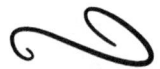

When life is busy and urgent needs are present, we need extra nutrients, sleep, and self-care—just like the tropical plants that soak in the sunlight and rain aplenty. And when conditions get colder, it's best to be still as we wait for the verdant spring to come again.

I have a huge-leafed tropical plant in my house. I also have fir trees. The two have nearly polar-opposite growing strategies, and it makes perfect sense, given the environments they would naturally grow in. Tropical plants are heat resistant, but they also consume a lot of available water. Having large leaves isn't a problem as long as the plants have a lot of water around and no worry of severe winters.

Fir trees, on the other hand, have extremely narrow needles that don't absorb nearly as much photosynthetic energy, and they don't use nearly as much water as tropical plants do when generating food. And since the species of fir trees in my house would normally encounter some colder temperatures and occasional snow (though not the deep winter colds or snows of areas away from the Pacific Northwest's somewhat more temperate climate), it's a great thing to have less photosynthesis going on. The fir trees need to reserve all of their nutrients and water until spring. They can't spend time worrying about growing leaves or vertical height.

Trees adapt to their environments rather than fight against the conditions they're given, and we can learn a lesson or two from the trees. So often, we try to have it both ways. Every day, we rush about, trying to pack in as much urgent stuff as we can, which causes stress and worry. We don't give ourselves the care we need to ensure that we have broad enough leaves to keep up our busy lifestyles. Then, when we do have downtime, when we could reserve our energy and recharge for the spring, like fir trees do, we feel anxious because it seems as though we're not doing enough. We are so used to moving at a certain clip that slowing down makes us anxious. So we pull out our phones and fill our valuable downtime with flurries of news feeds that often leave us feeling unfulfilled about ourselves and our world. We wonder why we feel imbalanced.

In our modern societies, we can't easily decide to be a broad-leafed tropical plant or a fir tree. Each of us has to deal with both scenarios. But we could adopt the strategies that each plant has developed over several million years in order to become successful in their environments.

When life is busy and urgent needs present themselves, we need extra nutrients, sleep, and self-care—just like the tropical plants that soak in the sunlight and rain aplenty. And when conditions get colder and nutrients are scarce, we need to focus on holding on and keeping one foot in front of the other. During those times, it's best to be still as we wait for the verdant spring to come again.

MINIMIZING MISSTEPS

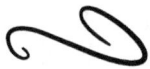

By preparing for missteps and disappointments, we not only stand a good chance of avoiding pitfalls, but also of minimizing the impact of our challenges so that we can spend more of our time and energy on the joy that each day brings.

The Forest Service has a number of JHAs or Job Hazard Analyses. The purpose of a JHA is to draw out the possible hazards that someone might encounter while performing a task such as trimming a tree or counting fish in a stream while snorkeling. People who are assigned these tasks sign off that they have reviewed the associated JHA. This process becomes somewhat routine, but it is based on a vitally important principle: we cannot control all the environmental factors out in the woods, but we need to control those we can while being attentive to the ones that are out of our control. That way, when a tree falls or a freak snowstorm hits, we are prepared for those impacts.

Going through the JHA process doesn't ensure that everybody who works in the woods will be one hundred percent safe all the time. But it does save lives and avoids injuries. Very few, if any, of those risks addressed by the JHAs are designed to help within the Forest Service headquarters or around our cars when we pull off to the side of the road to setup for a project. A JHA is designed specifically for the task we are doing.

Since JHAs focus so much on the dangers of tasks once people are on the job site, it can be easy to forget those risks when we're sitting comfortably in the office.

In similar ways, as human beings, we sometimes have a hard time giving enough headspace to the things we should watch out for in our daily lives. How easy is it to disregard dangers, disappointments, heartbreaks, or physical or emotional injury caused by the outside world when we are in the comfort of our homes, sipping a nice warm beverage as we view the sunrise. In that environment, all seems well with the world. If we're not careful—if we don't have some way to prepare for those riskier environments that we might face throughout the day—we will inevitably downplay the risks and only focus on the potential wins that the day might bring.

For me, writing things down makes those risks feel more permanent and present in my mind, so I take a few minutes while I'm in the comfortable environment of my kitchen with a beverage at hand to reflect on some ways I can mitigate those potential pitfalls and missteps. Then, when I face those scenarios, I won't have to think quite as hard about the best course of action because I will have already decided.

A few minutes of prep work, done each day and spread over several weeks, can add up to quite the shield against everyday disappointments as well as major emergencies. And let's face it, when we are in those challenging situations, our logical problem-solving brain is often hijacked by the more primitive survival side of our brain. That very preparation paid off for me in huge ways, one day, and allowed me to avoid a huge headache.

I had the chance to tag along with a wildlife biologist to film some wildlife in a very remote part of a forest for the day. We had a wonderful day, and I got a lot of great footage of animals and beautiful landscapes. When we got back to the truck and were loading our gear into the rig, I reached behind me as I took off my backpack. Only then did I realize something was missing. I checked my back pocket, and sure enough, my wallet wasn't there. My heart sank as I thought about all of the annoying tasks I would have to go through, from visiting the DMV to canceling and replacing credit cards. I told my wildlife-biologist coworker of my situation as a throw-away statement, quite certain we would never be able to find my wallet in that thick forest. Strangely enough, though, my coworker seemed confident that we'd find it if we retraced our steps. And within five minutes of walking back down the path we had taken that morning, we found my wallet lying on the path under a large log. It must have fallen out of my pocket as I climbed over the log.

I was amazed that we had found my wallet and was grateful for my coworker's brilliant navigational skills. I certainly wouldn't have been as confident in finding it as he was, let alone finding the right path. But my coworker explained that he has to clearly mark out when and where he goes long in advance so that he can conduct the right survey in the right section of the forest. He had planned out his trip down that particular path a year in advance and had mapped it all out well ahead of our time in the area.

I still think it was rather miraculous that I found my wallet, but I also understand why my friend was so confident that we would find it. He knew the exact path we had taken. Beyond the scientific need for a representative sample that necessitated visits to exact areas, it was important that my coworker be certain of when and where he was going. Especially for safety reasons, as he would spend most of his summers in the backwoods by himself.

In similar ways to JHAs, by preparing for missteps and disappointments, we not only stand a good chance of avoiding pitfalls, but also of minimizing the impact of those challenges that we have to deal with throughout our daily lives so that we can spend more time and energy on the joy each day brings.

THE ELEGANCE OF CREAM SODA AND A PINK COOKIE

A pink cookie and a can of red cream soda can make a few moments better, even when recovering from major brain injury.

I had my longest stretch of inpatient hospital care on a neuropediatric therapy unit when I was nine years old. The hospital was close enough that family visited me almost daily, but far enough away that it took serious sacrifices for them to do so. For instance, my family spent that Christmas in a RV on the hospital grounds. My hospitalization also pulled my parents' attention away from my siblings, who were young and definitely in need of their attention.

I'm so grateful for the support my siblings and parents gave me over those three months in the hospital.

But, for me, inpatient hospital-life generally had a sparse daily routine that consisted of little more than eating meals; going to physical, occupational, and speech therapy; sleep; and maybe a visit. Because of this, small traditions meant more to me than perhaps they did at any other time in my life. Receiving a custom-made T-shirt that was made especially for me by a favorite nurse. Getting a basketball from my neurosurgeon for Christmas. Having visits or sleepover parties with siblings. These were the things that made that hospital stay bearable, and in some respects, even enjoyable, at times.

And so it was with a routine that my dad and I developed over the months, a routine that neared sacred ritual status. For the first month and a half or so, I had to relearn how to walk and relied on a wheelchair most of the time. During that time, my dad would take me cruising around the hospital in the wheelchair, and the experience was so much a part of my experience there, that even thirty years later, I remember the color of the wallpaper and the way the evening sunlight slanted through the UV-film-coated windows of the walkway between the children's and adults' hospitals, which were connected by a bridge about a football field in length.

My dad would push me down the long corridor as I beat my hand against the armrest of the wheelchair to communicate. (I was also relearning how to talk.) My dad seemed to understand perfectly that I wanted to go as fast as I could and to feel the air rush past me, even if it was climate-controlled, filtered hospital air rather than fresh mountain gusts.

We'd then retrace our path back to the children's side, where two vending machines stood, and get a Fanta Red Cream soda with a Granny B's Pink Cookie (which always seemed too big and too delectable to purchase and eat for only fifty cents). We'd then park by the window and enjoy the sugar buzz as the sunlight faded.

Many of you might think this is a sad story about a boy with nothing but a cookie and a can of soda to look forward to, but I didn't feel picked on in those moments. I relished the sweetness of that cookie and the cool bite of that soda.

It's easy to overlay significant experiences with general emotional labels. But I've come to realize that, even in those desperate times when I felt more frustration and fear than any other time in my life, there were also moments of genuine goodness. Moments when I connected with remarkable friends and family and simple pleasures, like a cookie and a soda, could be made into vivid and enjoyable memories. So much so, that even though I haven't actually drunk a Fanta soda or eaten a Granny B cookie in decades, when I see them in vending machines, a smile creeps across my face.

In the darkest moments of life, I hope we can find moments of satisfaction, and yes, even joy. I found that a pink cookie and a can of red cream soda could make a few moments better, even during my recovery from a major brain injury, when I was in a wheelchair and unable to verbally express why those moments were important to me. We all have pink cookies to lighten the load of hard times. We just need to find them.

FILLING THE UNFORGIVING MINUTE WITH NURTURING SOIL & SUNLIGHT

We can find a way to forgive by recognizing that we all make mistakes from time to time.

Toward the end of the worst parts of the COVID-19 pandemic, I noticed an eighteen-inch eucalyptus tree that I'd been growing from a miniscule seed (and had been growing like crazy) was losing its leaves, shriveling fast. I jumped into action, gently repotting the seedling in a larger pot with rich compost and good nutrients and giving it a good drink.

Some people swoon about puppies. Well, I feel the same way about seedlings. I know—it's odd. Thus is my life. But those few days of watching one leaf after another fall or become crinkly was devastating for me. I planted the thing; I nurtured it from a seed into a real plant. And though I don't necessarily spend a lot of time on my seedlings' care, they do require consistent care, and this particular plant had been with me for most of the pandemic. It felt significant, somehow, because of that too.

Just when I was about to give up hope and deal with the prospect of starting over and planting a new seed (potentially waiting another two years for the new seedling to grow to the same extent), I saw a new leaf cluster forming on the main stem.

I was thrilled at so many levels. Most important, I would be able to watch as leaves grow back up the stem. And since the roots and stem remained healthy, I was hopeful the original seedling would make a full recovery.

Plants are rarely complicated. To care for a plant, we only need to do a few very simple things:

1. Plant the seed in good soil that is appropriate for the plant type.

2. Give it the right amount of sunlight for its species.

3. Water it sufficiently.

These three steps have nuances to them, and every plant species calls for a varying amount of the three elements, but assuming we know the right combination (which we can learn with a little research), and if we consistently follow these steps, we'll have healthy plants. Goodness knows, human relationships are not nearly as simple.

Since I knew the specifics and proper plant health for my little eucalyptus, I immediately knew I had missed a step or two. I decided that the seedling had outgrown its pot. Although I was watering the plant sufficiently, the amount of soil in the pot wasn't enough to retain the water the seedling needed to thrive between waterings. I'd put a strain on the plant every couple of days, forcing it to wait for its next watering until it finally reached a breaking point.

This discovery was useful to me, and it might be helpful to some aspiring gardeners out there. But I draw a deeper lesson from this experience. It made me grateful for second chances. For the chance to fix my mistake without permanent, devastating results. There are some actions we take in life that can't be undone as gracefully as I hope to have done with this seedling. But the experience with this plant reminded me of how many opportunities we have to give others and ourselves second chances. For instance, if someone says something unkind to me, I can write off the relationship entirely or, if the relationship matters to me, I can give it a second chance. When I'm not consistent with my Spanish lessons, yet again, I can give myself another chance.

When we give others additional chances, it doesn't mean that we disregard the hurt they caused or that we should open ourselves up to constant abuse.

Absolutely not!

Sometimes it is best to completely cut ties, especially when abuse is involved. But other times, we can find a way to forgive as we recognize the fact that we all make mistakes from time to time and that we all appreciate forgiveness. How wonderful it is that we can give that gift to others. Just like my eucalyptus seedling gave me a second shot and is doing a better job now that it receives appropriate care.

LEVERAGING HISTORY'S PERSPECTIVE

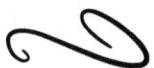

If we keep the broader perspective that history teaches us, we will feel assured that tomorrow will come and good things will happen in the future.

I had the great opportunity to study in England for a summer with a program affiliated with my master's degree. It was amazing to walk among nearly thousand-year-old buildings and know a bit about the history that those buildings have seen: wars, occupations, plagues, and political dynasties come and gone.

This immense historic timeline of the United Kingdom was particularly poignant when I visited Bath, which was a Roman resort town long before what we think of as England existed. During my visit, I took a tour of the bathhouse from which Bath gets its name, and I had the uncanny feeling that the space was timeless. It had been restored and maintained so well that they actually used it for public bathing up until the 1970s. That means the facilities served the same purpose for about two thousand years and served countless generations and lived through multiple government shifts. When I think of places like that, somehow, our current political crises feel less like end-of-the-world scenarios and more like challenging times we'll get through.

I try to put myself in the shoes of those who walked the cobblestone streets hundreds of years ago, and I try to think of the fears and hopes they felt. Our human desires haven't changed much. We still seek for growth, learning, happiness, and what is best for our families.

In fact, I'd dare say that the advancements in technology, life expectancy, and quality of life stem directly from a hope for a better life for ourselves and our families. Consider the push made in the United States to increase public services like plumbing and electrical systems in rural areas. We could take a cynical view on that effort, labeling it as a ploy to buy votes and gain political power, but those systems wouldn't have been put in place if local citizens from rural communities hadn't advocated and hoped for better public services.

Also consider the American public school system. While there is still room for improvement, when the system was first conceived, there was nothing like it in the world. The thought that every child would have the right to an appropriate education must have been extraordinary. It is rather amazing, even today.

When we consider the monumental events that have taken place throughout history, the importance placed on our daily fears, insecurities, and difficulties aren't minimized. In fact, we can take comfort in knowing that even in the most challenging of times, people still keep moving forward. The examples are in the past: Shop owners still baked bread during world wars. Waste management specialists still picked up trash during the recent pandemic.

If we keep that slice of hope and greater perspective in our minds, we will feel assured that tomorrow will come and good things will happen in the future. We will all face hard days, but just like those who lived before us came together and faced their challenges, we, too, will get through our tough times.

THE GIVING AND LIVING TREE

> Strive to grow as tall and as strong as possible. Don't cut yourself down with your thoughts or cut yourself short by refusing opportunities when they come.

Growing up in a somewhat arid part of the Intermountain West means that certain natural phenomena were foreign concepts to me when I first moved to the wet side of the Cascades in Oregon. So when I hiked with some of my Forest Service colleagues that first summer in town, I was blown away by what are called nurse logs.

Nurse logs are fallen trees or tree stumps that have young seedlings growing directly out of them.

As I walked around these amazing sprouts that grew directly out of the trunks of massive, old trees, it dawned on me what a perfect setup for success that was for the next generation of trees.

Forests with a lot of nurse logs tend to be wetter and denser than the forests I grew up hiking in. The canopies offer near-complete shade to the ground below. But seedlings rely on sunlight, like almost all trees, so without breaks in the canopy, there is little chance of new growth. When a mature tree falls, it leaves a gash of sunlight that can penetrate to the ground and nourish young saplings, which can grow inside the footprint of the mature tree.

As the old tree starts to decompose, it attracts micro-organisms that break down the woody material and then becomes excellent nutrients for the young trees. Consequently, the new generation of seedlings don't have to compete as fiercely with the mature trees that would otherwise block the sunlight, nor are they required to compete for water and nutrients.

There's a powerful lesson in the life cycle of these trees.

These trees grow as tall and as strong as they can while also providing habitat for a lot of biodiversity. In their vertical-growth period, they prioritize structural growth over things like seed production. This is vital because eventually that open space in the tree canopy will fill and successful saplings will have to be tall enough to reach the sunlight on their own. Once the trees have established healthy places in the canopy where they can absorb sunlight on their own, they shift to developing seeds and deepening roots. This allows them to withstand windstorms and other natural phenomena that can bring trees down.

Trees also rely on defensive strategies to keep bugs and diseases at bay. Some species use thick layers of bark to withstand wildfires. Others use sap to trap insects that might expose the trees to disease or other external attacks. Recent research has even found that trees communicate with other trees, notifying them of potential threats like bug infestations.[7]

Trees also naturally adapt to their current realities, rather than making rash decisions based on unrealistic expectations. During drought years, a tree's growth is much smaller than years when nutrients and water are plentiful. If we inspect a slice of a tree ring, we can easily see that difference.

In essence, trees take the long-run approach rather than the shorter and riskier approach to life that sometimes leads to huge rewards but can also be disastrous. By using these strategies and prioritizing their needs, some tree species can live for thousands of years. Even the grandest of trees have natural life expectancies. And when it's time for it to die, each tree gives space and nutrients to the earth so that the next generation of trees can thrive.

This concept teaches a subtle lesson. While we are living, we should truly *live*. We should strive to grow as tall and as strong as we can. We shouldn't cut ourselves down with our thoughts or cut ourselves short by refusing opportunities when they come. At the same time, when we, as mentors, teachers, and friends, can give space for others and encourage them to thrive, then we are laying new roots for ourselves and for future generations.

CHANGING OUR LIVES ONE HAIR CUT AT A TIME

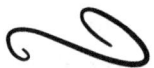

Just like getting your hair cut gives you the chance to look different, changing small things that you do each day can add up to extraordinary differences in your life.

Growing up, I always hating getting my hair cut. Not because the experience itself was unpleasant, but because I never liked the change in my appearance that the much shorter hair always seemed to bring. It always took a few weeks for my hair to grow back to an acceptable length and for me to feel comfortable again.

Now that I'm grown and can choose my own hairstyle, I am detailed in my vision before the cutting commences. I research different hairstyles that work well with different shapes of faces and sizes of heads, and I look up trends. I know—I'm a total geek. But to me, a positive change to my hairstyle makes as much of an impact on my overall look and my confidence and can do just as much as anything else to project my chosen style. It's important to me that I be excited about the result of my hair cut, especially since I only get my hair cut every couple of months. I don't want to dread looking in the mirror.

Appearances are definitely no measure of substance. We shouldn't judge the people around us as being smarter or more engaging or more world-wise or kinder or anything that may be based on their looks. In my personal living experience, I've noticed that when I *think* I look good and professional and presentable, I *feel* a bit better about myself. We shouldn't judge a book's contents by its cover, but the contents might feel a bit better about themselves when they are surrounded by the embrace of a beautiful cover.

When I was a teenager, I had a dear neighbor who was involved in a fundraiser for a nature center in town. My neighbor asked me to dress up in medieval-era clothes and become a wandering minstrel during the festival, which was geared around the summer solstice. I got a period-appropriate tunic and a rustic belt and sandals, and I got to carry a chicken puppet that was a hit with the kids.

Looking back, it is remarkable to me how easily and quickly I transformed into someone else. I even tried my hand at an English accent (with varying degrees of success) and spouted out Shakespearean soliloquies when asked to do so by the visiting public. Obviously, no one assumed I was a traveling minstrel from the sixteenth century, but realizing how easy it was to become a different person, makes me wonder if we could take a similar tactic with much smaller aspects of our lives.

Are there routines that we don't enjoy but we've been performing for so long that it hasn't dawned on us to change them? Do we feel we're in a rut that, in a real sense, keeps us from doing things that might bring greater joy into our lives? Maybe, upon some personal reflection, we realize that most weeks, we grit our teeth to make it through the work week and then dread Monday even when we still have two days of the weekend to enjoy.

Putting on the costume of the sixteenth-century English minstrel had some effect on me, sure, but playing the part helped me step into the role a whole lot better. And having people around me positively respond to my character helped even more. It was rewarding to see groups of kids let out a cheer when the chicken puppet let out a particularly convincing cluck.

At the end of the solstice event, when I regrettably took off the costume, I also gave up the character, but even now, so many years since, I tie a sense of self-worth and confidence to that experience. In a real sense, changing our outward appearance and taking on a slightly different character, can have an inward effect that is much deeper than the hairstyle we settle on or the clothes we wear.

Maybe we've wanted to take on a daily mindfulness routine or maybe we find ourselves dashing out the door without breakfast, which leads us to drag our feet toward irritability by early afternoon. Maybe we're always thinking about getting into better shape but the incumbent details are too overwhelming.

So we make a small change. Perform one task differently each week. Plan out our meals for the week. Take a short walk at lunchtime. Drink more water. What difference could those small changes make in our day?

Theater requires actors to imagine how a certain character would react according to the script's specified scenarios. What script would we like to write for our day? What role would bring meaning and joy? Trying out even a small role or a new routine in our life might just be the thing that liberates us from those ruts that so strongly hold us back. Just like getting our hair cut gives us the chance to look different, changing small daily tasks can add up to extraordinary differences in our life. And those small differences can ripple outward if we stick with them.

HERE'S THE REAL DEAL ON NEW YEAR'S RESOLUTIONS

Goal setting is designed to help us live more fulfilled lives, not add yet another thing that we feel like we ought to do because it's something good people ought to do.

One year, while growing up, my family and I each wrote down a few New Year's resolutions on small strips of paper. My mom was encouraging us to set some goals geared around how we could treat each other better as a family. We placed the strips of paper in a small wooden chest and were excited to see if we would accomplish our goals by the end of the next year when we would open the chest and review them. That chance never came. We either lost the chest or had other plans for the New Year's Eve celebrations the following year, so we didn't review our goals.

Making New Year's resolutions is a time-honored tradition, and I don't fault my mom at all for organizing the goal-setting activity. I'd imagine many of us relate to making such resolutions. "This year I'll lose those few extra pounds" or "I'll finally ask for that raise" or "I'm going to run that marathon." We tuck the slip of paper in a journal for safe keeping, and then, somehow, in a miraculous feat of time warping, we find that old scrap of paper with those hopeful aspirations at the close of yet another year.

There's nothing wrong with writing down and then setting aside our aspirations if our goal is to identify dreams that we'd like to remember from time to time. But if we actually want to attain our dreams throughout the new year, there are some simple ways to greatly improve our chances:

1. GOOD GOALS ARE ALWAYS WORKS IN PROGRESS. The goals that we actually achieve are kept at the top of our minds by identifying and performing tasks in small bites, little by little, day by day, and week by week.

    Thinking about all the work we'll have to put in to achieve our ultimate goals can be overwhelming. But if we break those goals into smaller, more digestible chunks, we can mark our progress, which helps to motivate us further. We can adjust our micro-goals for the day or week ahead based on our current difficulties and opportunities. By doing so, we avoid that sinking feeling that we'll never achieve such a massive goal because we're only looking at the portion that we are currently chipping away at.

    When I set out to write my first novel, I had no writing routine to build on and no idea what to do. Slowly, I picked up tips from friends who had published books, as well as from a lot of web searches and a couple of fabulous editors. But even when I had all the tricks of the trade in my head, I still needed to chip away at writing the manuscript page by page, day by day. That,

I discovered, is what keeps most people from publishing their novels. They just don't write consistently for a long enough time to finish their manuscripts. It's the same with any ambitious goal—we need to put in little infusions of time and effort each day that, in the long run, will lead to our success.

2. LESS IS MORE. I used to set dozens of detailed goals based on the different facets of life, from physical fitness to emotional wellness. Then I broke each goal down into seven or so categories. There's nothing wrong with being ambitious, but I've found that setting a few goals at a time works better than trying to accomplish everything at once.

    Instead, we might set monthly goals and focus on one facet of life at a time. Or we could create a prioritized list of goals so that, as we accomplish one goal, we know what our next focus will be.

3. WE ARE NOT MADE FOR GOALS; GOALS ARE MADE FOR US. Growing up, I was certain my elaborate goal-setting systems would impress others. And it did. People were impressed, but only setting goals doesn't help us become who we want to become or help us feel more fulfilled. That fulfillment comes from the changes in our lives that result from accomplishing worthwhile goals.

    Sometimes we focus so much effort on doing things the way we think effective people should, rather than focusing on what we personally need, that our goals get checked off lists but don't lead to the changes we want to see in our lives. If we spend more time thinking about who we want to be and what we want from life and less time worrying about word-smithing goals to sound impressive, we'll create more worthwhile goals to aspire to. And by focusing on the right goals, rather than jamming as many as we can into our lives or trying to impress others, we will be able to see positive changes.

The start of the New Year can be a powerful time to reset, re-evaluate, and forgive ourselves.

January 1 might be an arbitrary date on the calendar, but our brains know the difference between January 1 and January 8.

But some of the best ways to keep our goals alive takes more than the magic of a special day on the calendar. At the same time, giving ourselves grace when we don't quite reach our high aspirations is a wonderful thing. Few things kill hope faster than chastising ourselves for not measuring up.

It's important to remember that goal-setting is designed to help us live more fulfilled lives, not to create tasks that we ought to do because they are tasks that good people do.

So lets forgive ourselves when we don't live up to our high expectations. Question our shortcomings and investigate how to improve on our next attempt. Celebrate small steps forward, realizing that consistent, small gains add up to major positive shifts in our lives. Lets remind ourselves that we are all works in progress. Who knows what remarkable things we might accomplish if we keep our hope alive and motivation vibrant.

ENDNOTES:

1. 2023. *Species Factsheet: Sterna paradisaea.* Accessed March 9, 2023. http://datazone.birdlife.org/species/factsheet/arctic-tern-sterna-paradisaea.

2. Moran, Barbara. 2022. *Biologist behind "Song of the Humpback Whale' reflects on five decades since its release.* Radio Broadcast. WBUR. July 11. Accessed March 9, 2023. https://www.wbur.org/hereandnow/2022/07/11/5-years-songs-humpback-whale.

3. Armed Forces History Collections in cooperation with Public Inquiry Services, Smithsonian Institution. 2001. *Facts about the United States Flag.* September. Accessed March 9, 2023. https://www.si.edu/spotlight/flag-day/flag-facts.

4. 2021. *Flag Day: The History of Flag Day.* June 11. Accessed March 9, 2023. https://www.govinfo.gov/features/flag-day-2021.

5. 2021. *The Rescue.* Directed by E. Chai Vasarhelyi and Jimmy Chin. Produced by P.J. van Sandwijk, John Battsek, E. Chai Vasarhelyi and Jimmy Chin. National Geographic. Accessed March 9, 2023. https://films.nationalgeographic.com/the-rescue.

6. Darley, J.M., and C.D. Batson. 1973. ""From Jerusalem to Jericho": A study of situational and dispositional variables in helping behavior." *Journal of Personality and Social Psychology* 27 (1): 100-108. Accessed March 9, 2023. https://psycnet.apa.org/doiLanding?doi=10.1037%2Fh0034449.

7. Wohlleben, Peter. 2016. *The Hidden Life of Trees.* 8th. Vancouver: Greystone Books.

ABOUT THE AUTHOR

Chris Bentley is a District Ranger for the U.S. Forest Service. He received a Masters Degree from Indiana University's O'Neill School of Public and Environmental Affairs. He lives in the mountains of Southern Idaho where he enjoys jogging, hiking, and biking among the ponderosa pines.

Start a conversation or ask a question on his website: www.chrisbentleyinc.com or email: connect@chrisbentleyinc.com. You can also connect with Chris through social media:

Facebook: @cbentley1160
Instagram: @christoph.w.bentley
Twitter: @chris1bentley2"

www.ingramcontent.com/pod-product-compliance
Lightning Source LLC
Chambersburg PA
CBHW062209080426
42734CB00010B/1854